FORKS OVER KNIVES Flavor!

Also by Forks Over Knives

Forks Over Knives Family

The Forks Over Knives Plan

Forks Over Knives: The Cookbook

Forks Over Knives: The Plant-Based Way to Health

Delicious, Whole-Food, Plant-Based Recipes to Cook Every Day

FORKS OVER KNIVES Flavor!

Darshana Thacker with Carolynn Carreño

Preface by Brian Wendel

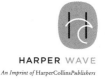

HARPER WAVE

An Imprint of HarperCollinsPublishers

HarperCollins books may be purchased for educational, business, or sales promotional use. For information, please e-mail the Special Markets Department at SPsales@harpercollins.com.

FIRST EDITION

Designed by Bonni Leon-Berman

Photography © 2018 Matt Armendariz Photography

Library of Congress Cataloging-in-Publication Data has been applied for.
ISBN 978-0-06-265276-8

20 21 22   GPS   10 9 8 7 6 5

Contents

FORKS OVER KNIVES Flavor!

Preface

by Brian Wendel, president of Forks Over Knives and creator and executive producer of the *Forks Over Knives* film

IT'S BEEN SEVEN YEARS since the launch of the feature film *Forks Over Knives*. I'm pleased to see a plant-based movement that's growing stronger each year, with more bloggers sharing recipes, more media coverage, and perhaps most exciting of all, more doctors recommending this way of eating for their patients suffering from chronic disease.

The film made the case that chronic ailments such as heart disease and type 2 diabetes can be prevented, halted, and oftentimes reversed by leaving animal-based foods and highly refined foods off the plate and adopt-

Living a life centered around food and cooking is something very dear to my heart. I grew up in Mumbai, India, with my father, one sister, one brother, and a mother who cooked for us three times a day. On a daily basis, my siblings and I spent time with Mom in the kitchen while she cooked and told us stories she invented for us. Every summer we spent a month as a family at my mom's childhood home, where her three uncles all lived with their wives and children. It was a large, sprawling house with a kitchen that was larger than most living rooms. There was no table and little counter space in the kitchen, so all of the work was done while sitting on the floor. From morning to night, my mom, the aunts, and the girl cousins in the house would sit together, chopping vegetables and rolling out chapati (Indian bread) on cutting boards, chatting and giggling while the women cooked on little coal burners that sat on the floor in the middle of the kitchen. Throughout the day, the men of the family and sometimes friends and neighbors, too, would come to the kitchen and sit down for meals that we had freshly prepared.

Looking back on my childhood, those hours spent in the kitchen were golden times. My life now is a world away, but those moments still inform my approach to cooking and food. Today my days are centered around the stove, much as my mom's were years ago. I cook almost every day, often all day. I frequently entertain friends and family over dinner, and I even occasionally find myself preparing the same dishes from those days in India. The recipes and the style of cooking may be different, but the experience of eating and sharing food with loved ones is very much the same.

From Vegetarian to a Whole-Food, Plant-Based Diet

I grew up in a Hindu, vegetarian family, so I have been intimately familiar with meals built around grains, beans, and vegetables from an early age. While being around the cooking of my mother and aunts taught me so much about vegetarian cooking, it wasn't until I was in my twenties that I started cooking myself.

During those twenty-something years, American TV arrived in Mumbai—and I soon became fascinated with the Food Network. I learned about various international foods and the multitude of ways in which meals can be prepared. After watching many, many hours of food shows, I decided I wanted to learn how to cook. So I adopted the cooking concepts I saw on television and applied them to vegetarian Indian cuisine. Using what I was learning on TV and the time spent in my family kitchen growing up, I began creating my own original recipes. My cooking career, you might say, had begun.

In 2001, I moved to the United States, and in 2003, I met Brian Wendel, the founder of Forks Over Knives, who told me he was a vegan. I had never heard the term, but Brian explained that this diet was one in which no animal products, including dairy and eggs, were consumed, and in which no animal was harmed or exploited in any way. I immediately thought, "Aha!" I knew, ethically, that that was the diet I had instinctively wanted to abide by all my life, and I immediately decided to give up all animal-derived foods.

In 2011, Brian made the *Forks Over Knives* film and asked me to cook for some early screenings of the film. At the time, I had my own small side business as a vegan caterer, and I taught classes in Indian vegan cooking. Through both watching the film and cooking the oil-free meals, I was introduced to the whole-food, plant-based lifestyle.

A whole-food, plant-based lifestyle is based on fruits, vegetables, whole grains, and legumes and excludes or minimizes meat, dairy products, and eggs, as well as highly refined foods such as bleached flour, refined sugar, and oil. The main energy sources in a plant-based diet are starches, in particular potatoes, sweet potatoes, whole grains, and legumes. Research has shown that by avoiding animal products and highly processed foods, we decrease our risk of developing common ailments, including heart disease, stroke, cancer, diabetes, and Alzheimer's disease.

Since my teen years, I had experimented with different ways of eating in specific components, to create your own inventions. For instance, the recipe for Huaraches: Mexican Masa "Flatbreads" with Beans and Lime-Spiked Salad (page 134), consists of various components: masa "cakes" shaped like *huaraches* (sandals), refried beans, salsa, and Tofu "Sour Cream" (page 334). These components can be reassembled to make other Mexican treats, such as tostadas, tacos, or a Mexican breakfast bowl with salsa and "sour cream" on top. The same concept applies to the various ethnic cuisines in the book. For instance, you can use the Thai Green Curry Paste that I use to make Thai Green Curry with Lima Beans (page 218) to re-create the classic Thai green curry with eggplant, green beans, and Thai basil. Or use the crust used for the Australian Pot Pie (page 229) to make a sweet or savory pie of your own creation.

One thing you will discover when you begin to enjoy whole-food, plant-based recipes is that you'll likely want to start cooking more. The food tastes great and leaves you feeling so good, you'll want to incorporate more and more of it into your life. Brian and I eat the majority of our meals at home; we almost always bring homemade food to the office, and we also entertain often at home. In order to make cooking as easy as possible, I have developed some habits and routines for preparing homemade meals on the go.

So read on as I give you a tour of my kitchen, showing you what I keep on hand and how I prepare myself so that cooking is as simple and enjoyable as possible, and share with you my favorite recipes from every corner of the globe.

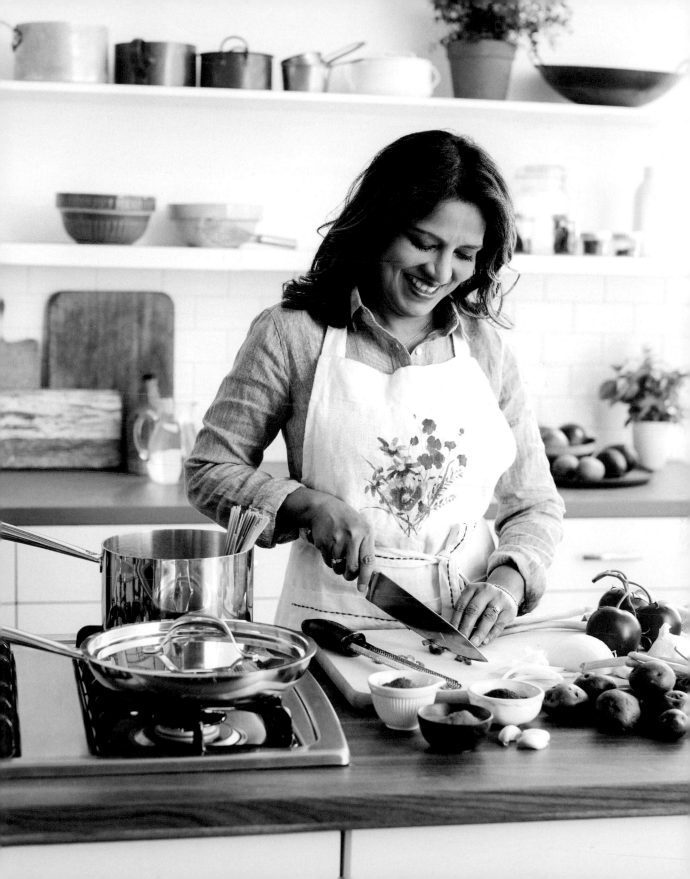

Having a well-stocked kitchen makes easy work of preparing healthy, tasty food. Think of these recipes as building blocks. Keep them in the refrigerator or freezer and you will see how simple it can be to cook a plant-based diet.

Essentials

Stocking a Whole-Food, Plant-Based Kitchen

Below are lists, by category, of the ingredients I keep in my house at all times. These include dry goods, refrigerated staples, such as condiments, and a freezer packed with frozen vegetables, beans, and grains that allow me to put together breakfast, lunch, and dinner on a daily basis with ease.

Dried Herbs and Spices

I rely on dried herbs and spices to add layers of flavor and nuance to just about everything I make, including soups, sauces, and dressings. The following are the dried herbs and spices I use and that I suggest you stock.

Allspice (ground)

Basil

Bay leaves

Black pepper (ground)

Cayenne

Cinnamon (ground sticks)

Chile powder (ancho, árbol, chipotle, New Mexico, and pasilla)

Caraway (seeds and ground)

Cloves (whole and ground)

Coriander (seeds and ground)

Cumin (seeds and ground)

Fennel (ground)

Fenugreek (ground)

Galangal (ground)

Garlic powder

Kaffir lime (ground)

Lemongrass (ground)

Marjoram

Nutmeg (ground)

Onion powder

Oregano (Mexican and regular)

Parsley

Red pepper flakes

Rosemary

Sage

Star anise (whole)

Paprika (sweet and smoked)

Sumac (ground)

Tarragon

Thyme

Turmeric (ground)

White pepper (ground)

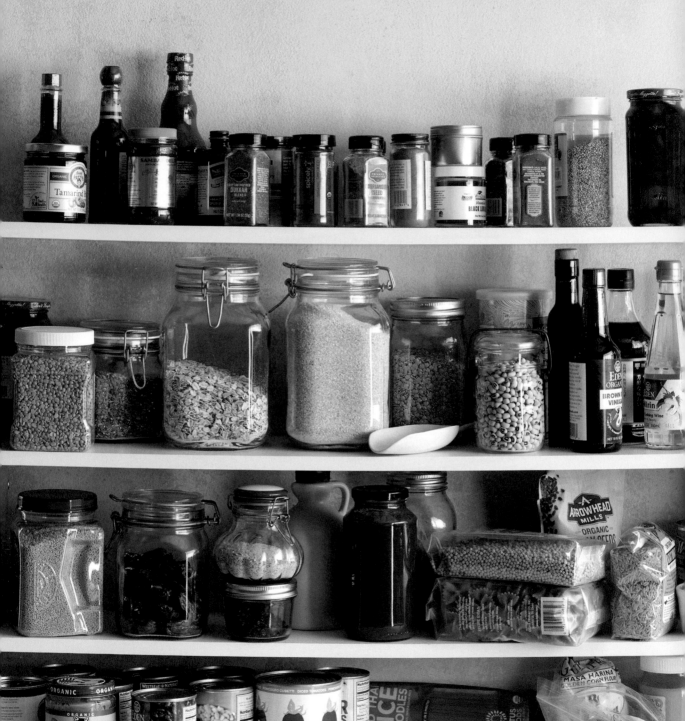

SPICE BLENDS

Many cultures have a signature blend of spices that allow you to add a combination of herbs and spices to a dish at one time. I make my own blends when they are made from ingredients I have on hand, so I can make them to my liking, or when I think the blend may not be readily available. These are some that I use often.

Berbere spice blend, also called Ethiopian spice blend, consists primarily of paprika, with other seasonings from fenugreek and garlic to cloves, cinnamon, and allspice. You can use garam masala in its place. For my homemade version of Berbere Spice Blend, see page 204.

Cajun spice blend, a blend of paprika, black pepper, cumin, fennel seed, and dried herbs used in Louisiana Vegetable Gumbo (page 199) and any dish in which you want Cajun flavor. I make my own, but you can also use a store-bought blend. For my homemade version of Cajun Spice Blend, see page 151.

Five-spice powder, a mix of ground star anise, cloves, cinnamon, Sichuan pepper, and fennel seed, five-spice powder, often called "Chinese five-spice powder" adds a distinctly Chinese flavor to sautés and sauces.

Garam masala, a popular Indian spice blend that includes cumin, coriander, cardamom, pepper, cinnamon, cloves, and nutmeg.

Italian seasoning, which quickly adds flavors of Italy; this blend contains basil, marjoram, oregano, rosemary, thyme, and garlic.

Ras el hanout, a North African spice blend. I make my own because it is made with spices, including coriander, paprika, turmeric, and cinnamon, that I always have on hand. For my homemade version of Ras el Hanout, see page 188.

Togarashi, a spicy Japanese spice blend of chiles, nori, sesame seeds, and orange peel.

Bulgur Cracked wheat best known for its role in tabbouleh.

Couscous and Israeli couscous Couscous is a tiny pasta that feels like a grain. Israeli couscous is larger and chewier.

Farro A chewy Italian grain and member of the wheat family. Other hearty berries such as wheat berries, barley, spelt, or rye berries may be used in its place.

Flaxseeds (meal and whole) Flax meal is ground flaxseeds. I use it to make a wash, which I brush on all my pastries before baking them. Similar to an egg wash in conventional baking, a flaxseed wash helps pastry brown beautifully. I also use it in baked goods.

Freekeh Middle Eastern smoked cracked wheat. Use it interchangeably with bulgur.

Millet A mild-tasting gluten-free grain common in India and North Africa.

Oats (rolled and steel-cut) Steel-cut oats are whole oat groats that have been chopped. Rolled oats are pressed and cook significantly more quickly.

Quinoa A gluten-free grain and the grain I use most other than rice.

Rice (short-grain, long-grain, Thai red rice) I keep a variety on hand. Short-grain rice is chewier and more glutinous.

Sorghum A chewy, round, gluten-free grain that is great in salads and soups.

NUTS AND SEEDS

I keep a variety of nuts and seeds, and a few nut and seed butters in my fridge. I occasionally include nuts and seeds in baked goods or salads. Sometimes I use the butters to make sauces or dressings, such as Peanut Sauce (page 337) and Indonesian Peanut Sauce (page 114).

Almonds (whole almonds and almond butter)

Cashews I use cashews in many recipes to give a creamy texture. Because of their mild flavor, they are ideal for making "cream" and "cheese."

Peanuts (roasted peanuts and peanut butter) Peanuts and peanut butter have a very distinct flavor, so I tend to use them sparingly, generally where they are traditionally used, such as in Southeast Asian cuisine.

Pecans I like sweet, nutty pecans in both salads and desserts.

Pistachios Toasting really brings out the flavor of pistachios, and they're easy to find in grocery stores. I use pistachios primarily in desserts.

Poppy seeds I like the crunch that poppy seeds bring to breads and sweet baked goods.

Pumpkin seeds have a distinct, delicious flavor. I use them in breads, salads, and desserts. I buy toasted pumpkin seeds, but they are also easy to toast in the oven, following any recipe for toasted nuts.

Sesame Seeds (toasted seeds and tahini) Toasted seeds have so much more flavor than raw; you can find them in a shaker canister in the Japanese section of grocery stores. They're delicious sprinkled on salads and any Asian dishes. Sesame butter (or tahini) is a delicious base for dressings and sauces, and it is the foundation of hummus.

Walnuts I use walnuts to make pie crusts and in other baked goods.

PASTA AND NOODLES

I keep a variety of pasta and noodles on hand, including Thai-style brown rice noodles, brown rice, quinoa, and whole-wheat Italian pasta in various shapes, and Japanese buckwheat noodles (called soba noodles) and udon noodles.

PLANT MILK

I give you a recipe for homemade almond milk, but if you choose to buy plant milk instead, look for brands with as few ingredients as possible, such as West-to soups, stews, and cooked vegetables. Use fresh herbs as a garnish.

Leafy greens (fresh lettuce, spinach, and kale, and other greens in bunches): Wash, dry, and store in a plastic bag with a paper towel. Refrigerate for up to 5 days.

Lemon and lime juice Squeeze in large quantities using an electric or handheld juicer; refrigerate for up to 10 days or freeze for up to 1 month.

Onion Chop by hand; refrigerate or freeze in 1-cup portions. It is not necessary to thaw the onion before cooking.

Potatoes, sweet potatoes, and yams Steam or bake and refrigerate in airtight containers.

Seasonal vegetables Trim and cut green beans, and cut cauliflower and/or broccoli into florets. Refrigerate for up to 1 week or freeze for up to 1 month. Also, if you have fresh vegetables that may go bad before you use them, whether mushrooms, bell peppers, zucchini, scallions, you name it, chop them, put them into zip-top bags, and freeze for up to 1 month; no need to thaw before cooking.

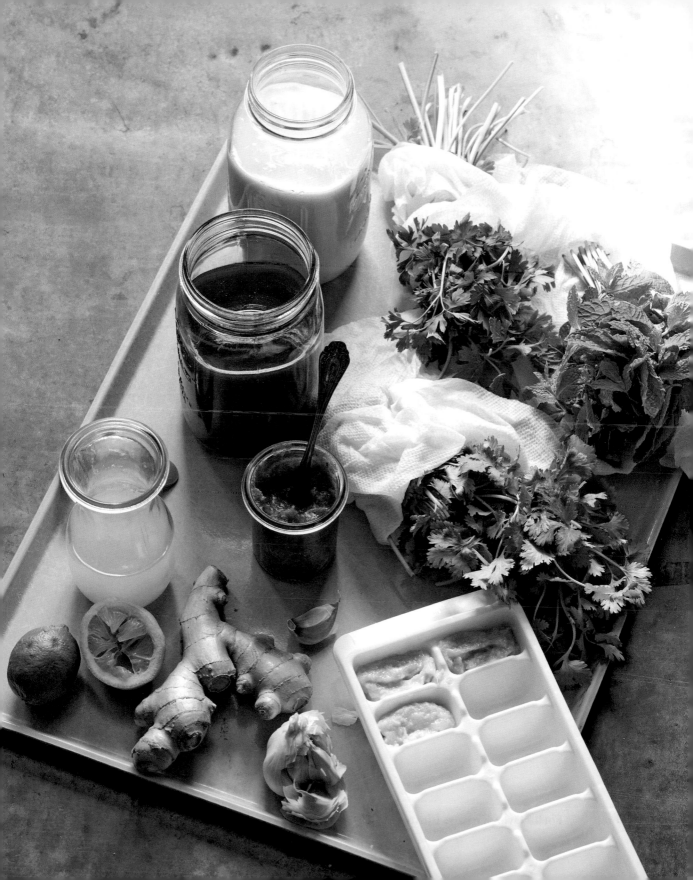

Myrna's Marinara Sauce

Makes about
4 cups

Ready in
40 minutes

When Brian and I visit his mom, Myrna Wendel, in Florida, she often makes her delicious marinara sauce because she knows how much we like it. She shared her recipe with me, and I could hardly believe how simple it was to make. There is virtually no prep work: you just throw all the ingredients into a pot, bring it all to a simmer, and, half an hour later, your thick, rich tomato sauce is ready. I use it to make Spaghetti Tricolore with Myrna's Marinara Sauce (page 252), Zucchini Rollatini Stuffed with Quinoa and Chickpeas (page 232), Crispy Polenta Sticks with Spicy Marinara Sauce (page 80), Sicilian Rice Balls with Mushroom and Peas (page 85), and Rustic Pizza Toasts (page 88). I also keep it on hand to make a quick, simple last-minute pasta dinner.

1½ pounds ripe, red tomatoes, seeded and chopped (about 3½ cups)

1 (28-ounce) can sodium-free or low-sodium crushed tomatoes

8 garlic cloves, roughly chopped (about 3 tablespoons)

4 pitted dates, chopped (about 2½ tablespoons)

¼ teaspoon freshly ground black pepper

Sea salt

¼ cup chopped fresh basil

1. In a large pot, combine the chopped tomatoes, canned crushed tomatoes, garlic, dates, and pepper and bring to a boil over high heat. Reduce the heat to medium-low and simmer, uncovered, for about 30 minutes, stirring occasionally.

2. Turn off the heat and use an immersion blender to puree the tomatoes into a sauce. Add salt to taste and stir in the basil leaves.

STORAGE: Cool to room temperature and transfer the sauce to a container with a tight-fitting lid. Refrigerate for up to 1 week or freeze for up to 1 month.

Cashew Chickpea "Cheese"

I use a combination of cashews and chickpeas to make this creamy, delicious vegan cheese. To firm up the "cheese," I use agar-agar, which is a natural gelatin derived from seaweed. If I will be grating the cheese, I freeze it, which gives it a hard, grated consistency. I add this cheese to Twice-Baked New Potatoes with Cashew Chickpea "Cheese" (page 95), Polenta Pizza with Summer Garden Vegetables (page 147), Penne with Eggplant-Lentil "Bolognese" Sauce (page 248), and Mushroom and Kale Farrotto (page 280). Use it anywhere that grated cheese would be welcome.

Makes about 1 cup

Ready in 1 hour

½ cup raw cashews

¼ teaspoon agar-agar (or ½ teaspoon agar-agar flakes)

½ (15-ounce) can chickpeas, drained and rinsed (about ¾ cup)

3 tablespoons nutritional yeast

1 tablespoon fresh lemon juice

1 tablespoon light miso paste

½ teaspoon Italian seasoning

Sea salt

Freshly ground black pepper

1. Line a medium ramekin or muffin cup with plastic wrap.

2. Soak the cashews in ¾ cup hot water for 15 minutes. Drain.

3. Combine the agar-agar and ⅓ cup water in a medium saucepan and bring to a boil over high heat. Reduce the heat to medium-low and simmer, stirring constantly with a spoon, for 5 to 7 minutes, until the agar-agar granules have dissolved. To test, lift the spoon out of the pot and let it cool for a few seconds; touch the spoon to feel for granules. If the spoon feels grainy, simmer for another minute and test it again.

4. Combine the cashews, chickpeas, nutritional yeast, lemon juice, miso, Italian seasoning, and agar-agar water in a blender or food processor and pulse to a smooth paste. Add salt and pepper to taste.

5. Spoon the "cheese" spread into the prepared ramekin with a rubber spatula. Chill in the freezer for 45 minutes or in the refrigerator for at least 2 hours, until the "cheese" is firm.

6. To use, turn the ramekin over onto a serving plate and tap the bottom of the ramekin to slide the spread out onto the plate. Pull off and discard the plastic wrap. Serve the "cheese" as a dip with crudités or toasted pita chips.

STORAGE: Refrigerate, covered, for up to 1 week or freeze for up to 1 month.

What you eat for breakfast informs how you feel physically and emotionally all day long. Whether it's a healthy, hearty bowl of savory goodness or a sweet breakfast treat, start your day with a meal that leaves you feeling like it's going to be the best day ever!

1 | Breakfast

for about another 4 minutes, until golden brown. Line a bowl with a dishcloth and place the tortillas in the bowl. Cover with the cloth to keep the tortillas warm until you're ready to use them. Repeat, cooking the remaining tortillas in the same way.

4. Preheat a large nonstick sauté pan over medium-high heat. Lay the plantain slices in the sauté pan and cook for 3 to 4 minutes, until the undersides are caramelized. Flip and cook for another 3 to 4 minutes, until caramelized. Remove the plantains from the sauté pan and set aside.

5. Combine the beans, half of the cilantro, the cumin, and ½ cup water in a large sauté pan and cook them over medium heat for about 5 minutes, smashing the beans with a potato masher, until they are warmed through.

6. To serve, place one tortilla on a plate and spread the beans over them. Top with a few slices of plantains and a dollop of "sour cream." Garnish with the remaining cilantro and serve warm. Repeat, building the remaining tortillas in the same way.

STORAGE: Refrigerate the cakes in a covered container or sealable plastic bag for up to 5 days or freeze for up to 1 month. Warm them in a 350°F oven before serving. Serve with freshly made toppings.

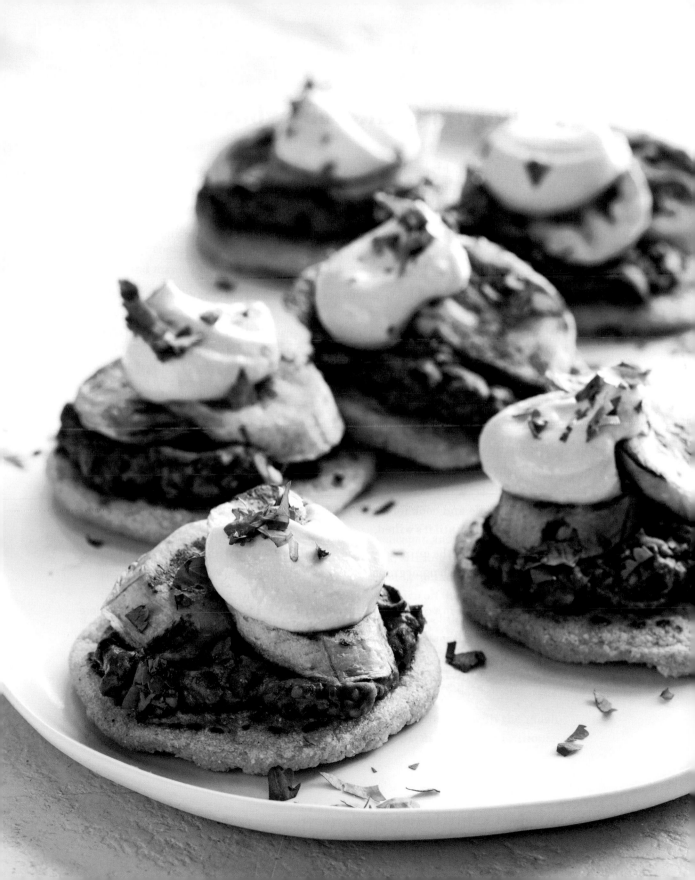

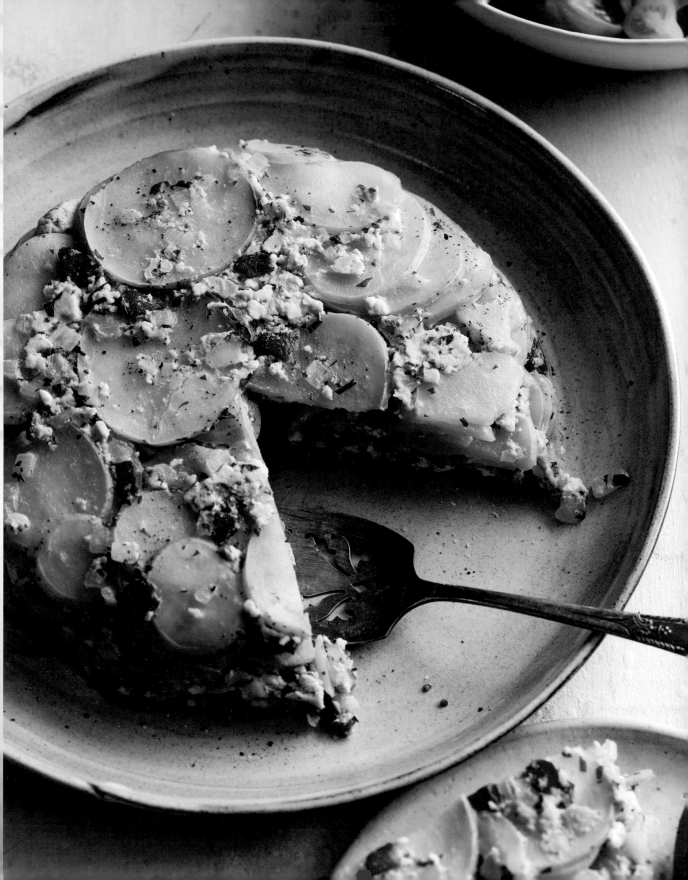

Tortilla Española with Potatoes and Sweet Red Peppers

A Spanish tortilla is an egg-based dish, similar to a frittata. (It bears no resemblance to a Mexican tortilla.) Spanish tortillas are traditionally eaten as an appetizer, but I like them for breakfast. I find something romantic about serving a tortilla Española to brunch guests, maybe because I know the care that went into preparing it. This tortilla tastes great reheated, so it's a good dish to make in advance for a brunch or party.

Makes 1 10-inch tortilla

Ready in 1 hour, 15 minutes

NOTE: Aquafaba is the liquid left over when cooking beans (usually chickpeas). It is often used in vegan cooking as a binder in place of eggs. You can also use the canning liquid from canned beans.

NOTE: You will need a 10-inch pie dish to make this.

2 pounds Yukon Gold potatoes, scrubbed and thinly sliced (about 8 cups)

7 ounces extra-firm tofu, drained and finely crumbled (1 cup)

¼ cup plus 2 tablespoons aquafaba (liquid from canned or cooked beans)

2 tablespoons unbleached all-purpose flour (or whole-wheat flour)

1 tablespoon chickpea flour

⅛ teaspoon ground turmeric

1 medium yellow onion, cut into ¼-inch dice (about 2 cups)

2 medium garlic cloves, minced (about 1 teaspoon)

½ cup (½-inch diced) jarred roasted red bell peppers

3 tablespoons finely chopped fresh parsley

½ teaspoon black salt (or sea salt)

Freshly ground black pepper

1. Preheat the oven to 425°F. Line a 10-inch pie dish with parchment paper.
2. Place a steamer basket in a medium saucepan and add 1 to 2 inches of water to the pan. Bring the water to a simmer over medium-high heat. Place the potatoes in the steamer, cover, and steam until tender when pierced with a fork, about 15 minutes. Transfer the potatoes to a large bowl and set aside.

4. Preheat a nonstick sauté pan over medium-low heat for 3 minutes, or until a drop of water dances when it hits the pan. Pour ⅓ cup of the batter in the center of the pan and use a crepe spreader or an offset spatula to spread the batter into a thin 5-inch round. Cook for 2 to 3 minutes, until the undersides are lightly browned. Use a thin spatula to turn the pancakes and cook for 2 to 3 minutes, until golden brown on the second side. Place the pancakes on a baking sheet and cover with a cloth or place in a 200°F oven to keep warm while you make the remaining pancakes.

5. Serve warm with the topping of your choice.

STORAGE: Place the pancakes in a covered container or sealable plastic bag and refrigerate for up to 5 days or freeze for up to 1 month. Warm them in a 300°F oven until they are heated through.

Maple Orange Sauce

Makes about
1½ cups

Ready in
15 minutes

2 tablespoons raw cashews

2 tablespoons pure maple syrup

1 teaspoon orange zest

1 orange, peeled and seeded, cut into 1-inch pieces (about ¾ cup)

1. Soak the cashews in ½ cup hot water for 10 minutes.

2. Transfer the cashews and soaking water to a blender. Add the maple syrup, orange zest, and chopped orange and blend into a smooth sauce.

STORAGE: Refrigerate in a covered container for up to 1 week.

Banana Chocolate Sauce

Makes about
1½ cups

Ready in
5 minutes

2 bananas, cut into large pieces

¾ cup almond milk

¼ cup plus 1 tablespoon cocoa powder

2 tablespoons Date Paste (page 30)

⅛ teaspoon pure vanilla extract

Combine the bananas, almond milk, cocoa powder, date paste, and vanilla in a blender and blend until smooth.

STORAGE: Refrigerate in a covered container for up to 1 week.

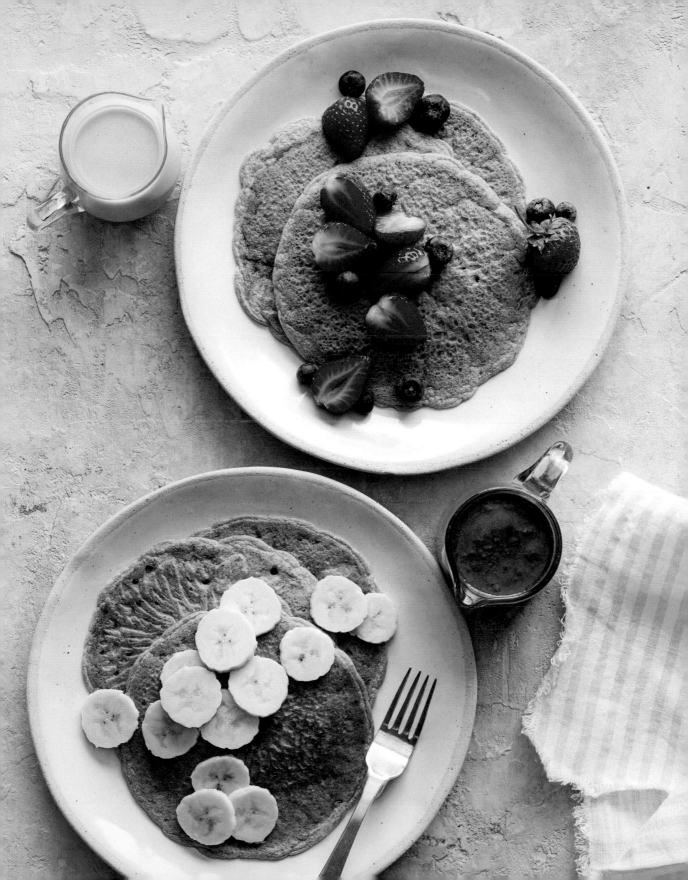

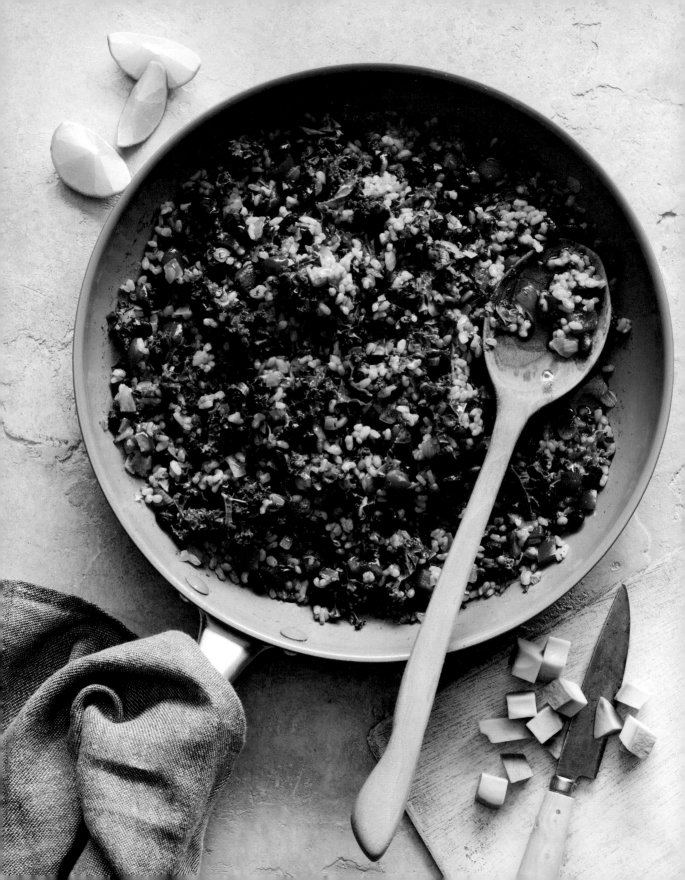

Gallo Pinto: Costa Rican Breakfast Bowl

Gallo pinto is a popular Costa Rican breakfast dish of black beans and rice. Brian's brother Josh, who lives and owns a café in Costa Rica, is known for his version of gallo pinto. I asked Josh for his recipe, and I was happy to discover that it's as simple to make as it is tasty. I start with left-over rice and canned beans, which makes this recipe quick and easy to throw together when I start the day.

Makes about
4 cups

Ready in
20 minutes

½ yellow onion, cut into ¼-inch dice (about 1 cup)

1 medium red bell pepper, cored, seeded, and cut into ½-inch dice (about 1 cup)

1 teaspoon ground cumin

1 teaspoon garlic powder

½ jalapeño pepper, seeded and minced (optional)

½ bunch kale, stems removed and discarded, leaves shredded (about 2 cups)

2 cups cooked short- or long-grain brown rice (from about ⅔ cup uncooked rice)

1 (15-ounce) can black beans, rinsed and drained (about 1½ cups)

3 tablespoons finely chopped fresh cilantro

Sea salt

1 avocado, cut into ½ inch dice

1 lime, cut into wedges

1. Combine the onion, bell pepper, cumin, garlic powder, and jalapeño (if you're using it) in a large sauté pan. Add ½ cup water and sauté the vegetables over medium heat for about 10 minutes, until they are tender, stirring occasionally and adding 1 to 2 more table-spoons water as needed to prevent the vegetables from sticking to the pan. Add the kale, rice, beans, and 1 cup water and cook over medium heat for 3 to 5 minutes, folding the ingredients, until the kale has wilted and the liquid has been absorbed.

2. Add half of the cilantro and salt to taste and stir to combine. Garnish with the remaining cilantro and serve with diced avocado on top and a lime wedge.

"When a recipe calls for half of an onion, dice the other half, put it in a sealable plastic bag, and freeze it for use in another recipe. There is no need to thaw the onion before adding it to a sauté pan."

Playfulness is what defines appetizers, from finger foods, dips, and things to be dipped, to miniature versions of classics and snacks that date back to our childhoods. But who says you can't fill up on appetizers, especially nutritious options like those you'll find here?

2 | Appetizers

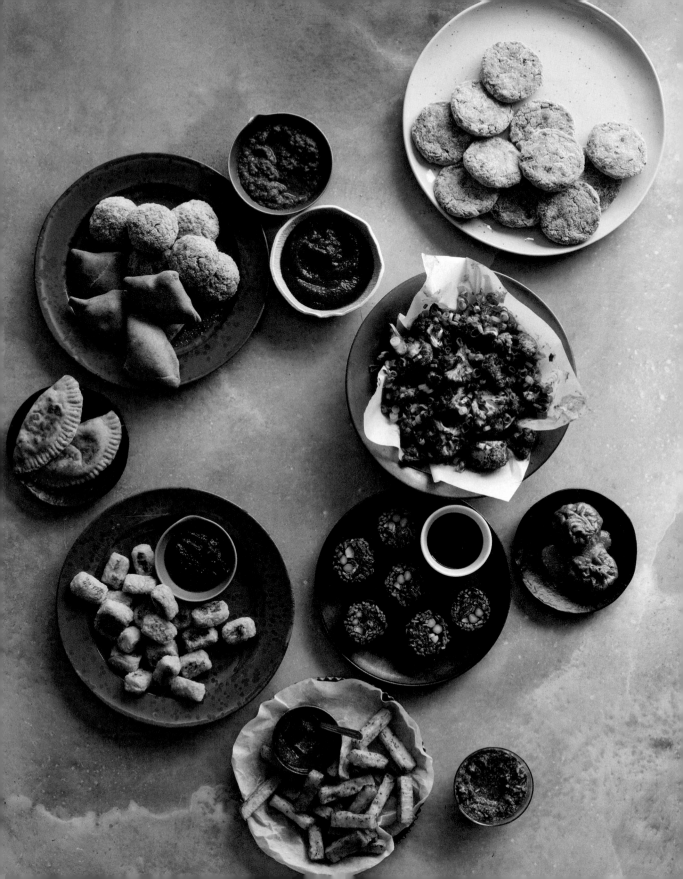

Corn and Mushroom Empanadas with Chimichurri

Empanadas are single-serving pastries that can be filled with sweet or savory ingredients. They are made in many parts of the world, but they are especially identified with Argentina. Empanadas are traditionally fried, but these are baked. The combination of potato flour and whole-wheat flour gives the pastry a light, crisp texture. I serve the empanadas with Chimichurri (page 340), a traditional Argentinian herb-based condiment. Empanadas are labor-intensive, but you can prepare the dough and filling, and even assemble them, a day in advance. Then all you'll have to do is bake them just before serving.

Ready in 3 hours

Makes 24 to 30 empanadas

NOTE: If you can't find potato flour, use 1½ cups mashed, cooked russet potatoes (about 1½ pounds) instead.

For the Dough
½ cup raw cashews

1 cup potato flour

½ cup whole-wheat flour

½ teaspoon sea salt

Unbleached all-purpose flour (or whole-wheat flour) for dusting

For the Filling
½ pound white mushrooms, trimmed and roughly chopped (about 3 cups)

1 small yellow onion, cut into ¼-inch dice (about 1 cup)

1 jalapeño pepper, seeded and finely chopped (about ¼ cup)

2 medium garlic cloves, minced (about 1 teaspoon)

3 cups fresh or frozen corn kernels (from about 3 large cobs)

2 tablespoons white miso paste

2 teaspoons ground cumin

¼ teaspoon cayenne pepper

¼ teaspoon freshly ground black or white pepper

3 cups fresh spinach (about 3 ounces), chopped

Sea salt

1 cup finely chopped fresh cilantro

1 tablespoon flaxseed meal (brown or golden)

Chimichurri (page 340)

minutes, until the leek is soft, stirring occasionally and adding 1 to 2 tablespoons water as needed.

4. Add the green beans, peas, cumin, coriander, garam masala, and ¼ cup water; cover and cook for about 10 minutes over medium heat, until the vegetables are tender, stirring occasionally and adding 1 to 2 more tablespoons of water as needed to keep the vegetables from sticking to the pan.

5. Transfer the vegetables to the bowl containing the potatoes. Add 1 cup of the ground puffed rice, the lime juice, cilantro, and salt and pepper to taste and stir to combine. The mixture needs to be dry enough to form into a patty; if it is too moist, add more puffed rice to achieve the correct consistency.

6. Dust your palms with cornmeal. Scoop up ¼ cup of the sweet potato mixture and form into a ball. Roll the ball in the cornmeal, making sure it is entirely covered, and press it into a flat patty. Place the patty on the prepared baking sheet. Continue forming the remaining tikkis in the same way. (If you are making the tikkis in advance, place them in a sealable plastic bag and refrigerate them for up to 3 days or freeze for up to 1 month.)

7. Bake the tikkis in the oven for 20 to 25 minutes, until the underside is golden brown and slightly crispy. Remove the baking sheet and turn each patty with a spatula. Return them to the oven and bake on the second side for 20 to 25 minutes.

8. Serve warm with fresh cilantro chutney or Nepalese tomato chutney on the side.

STORAGE: Refrigerate the baked tikkis for up to 1 week or freeze for up to 1 month. Warm them in a preheated 350°F oven until they are heated through. If you have refrigerated or frozen the tikkis before baking, bake them according to the recipe, adding about 5 minutes per side for frozen tikkis.

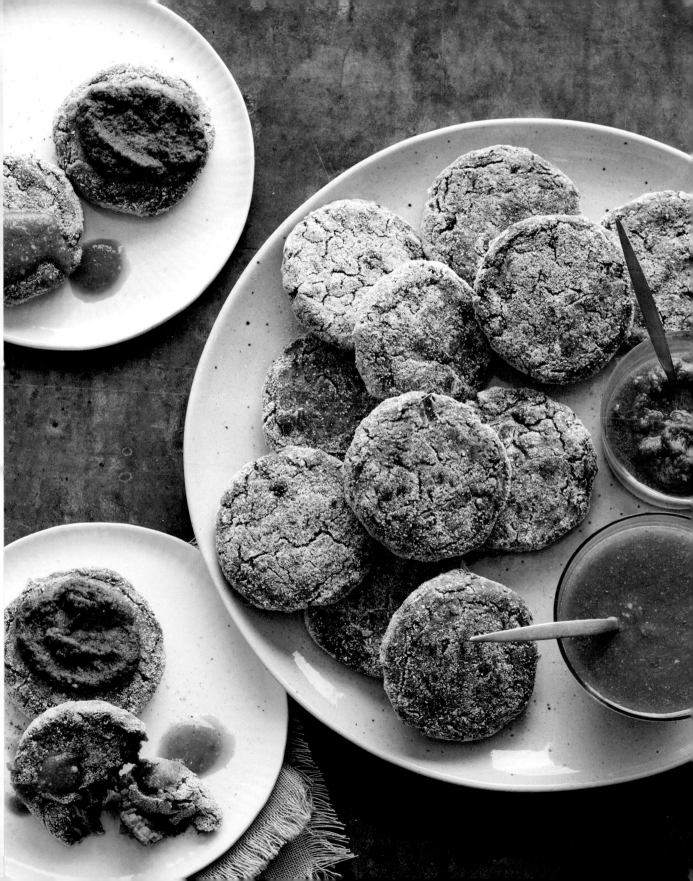

fingers in the water as you spread the rice; this will keep the rice from sticking to your fingers.

5. Lay the cucumber, asparagus, and pickled vegetables on the rice, making sure each vegetable is represented along the length of the sushi so you get each flavor in every bite of the sushi roll.

6. Lift the bottom edge of the mat and roll the nori sheet over the vegetables, making sure to tuck the veggies under as you roll so they are not pushed out the back side. Roll the sealed edge along the cutting board to seal it closed. Press the open ends to pack in any rice and vegetables trying to escape the sides.

7. Dip a long, sharp knife in the bowl of water and use it to cut the roll in half. Cut each half in half again and then again, until you have eight cut pieces.

8. Repeat with the remaining rolls. Serve with tamari for dipping.

Quick Vegetable Pickle

Makes about
2 cups

Ready in 3 hours

Pickling has been used around the world for centuries as a way to preserve vegetables. I have adopted traditional pickling vegetable methods from cultures where vinegar is used instead of oil. These include American coleslaw, Salvadoran curtido, German sauerkraut, and Korean kimchi, all of which are or can easily be made oil-free, vegan, and low in salt. This recipe for a quick pickled salad is ready in a few hours and lasts for up to a month in the refrigerator. I always have some on hand to add to salads, wraps, and tacos. It is an integral component of Red Rice Sushi Rolls (recipe above). Technically the vegetables are ready after three hours, but for best results, allow them to rest in the pickling liquid for a day or two before using them.

2 cups shredded red cabbage (about 8 ounces)

1 cup shredded Napa cabbage (about 3 ounces; or Savoy or green cabbage)

1 carrot, peeled and grated on the largest holes of a box grater (about ½ cup)

¼ cup fresh lemon juice

¼ cup brown rice vinegar

¼ teaspoon sea salt (optional)

Combine the ingredients in a large bowl and gently massage the pickling ingredients into the vegetables for a few minutes; this helps the vegetables break down. Transfer the vegetables along with the liquid to a clean jar with a tight-fitting lid. Refrigerate for at least 3 hours and ideally 2 days before using.

STORAGE: Refrigerate in a container with a tight-fitting lid for up to 1 month.

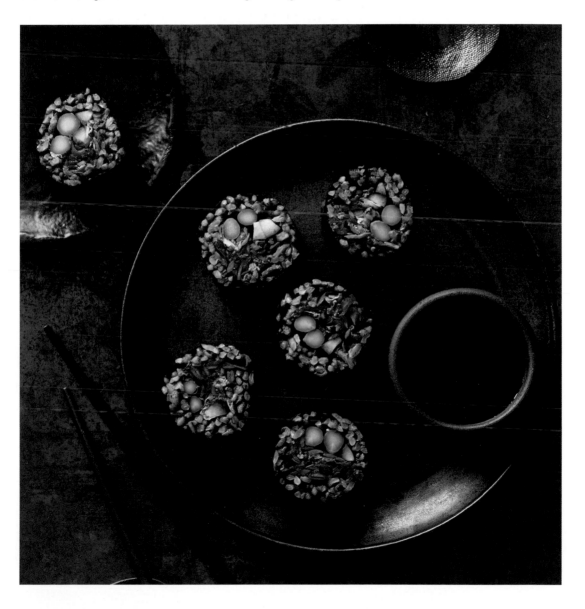

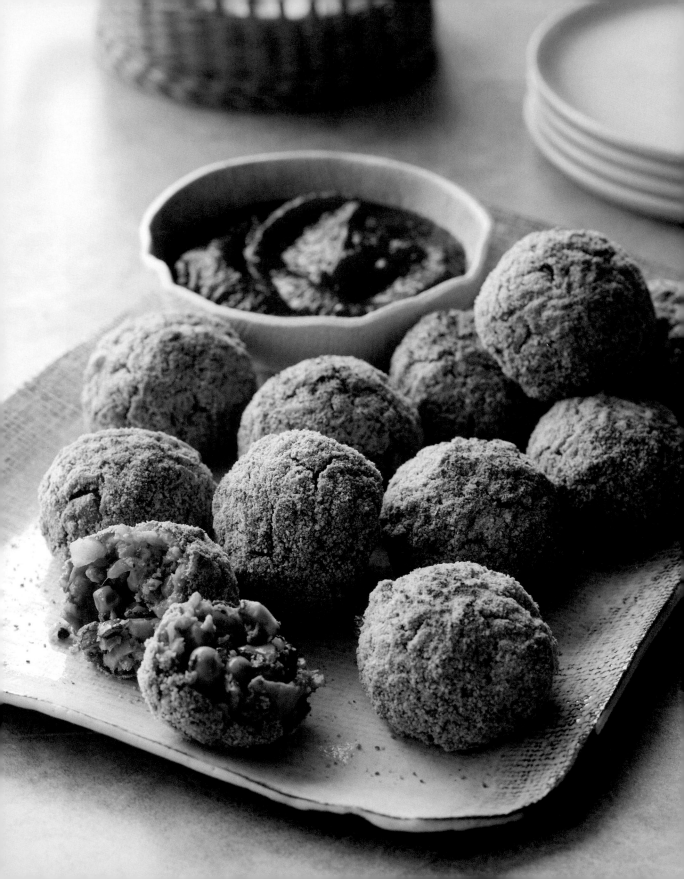

Sicilian Rice Balls with Mushrooms and Peas

Rice balls, known as *arancini* in Italy, are a Sicilian snack of leftover cooked rice mixed with other flavorful ingredients (usually meat sauce), breaded, and deep fried. The balls are so popular, you find them on display in just about every bar and train station in Sicily. I stuff these arancini with a ragù of mushrooms and green peas, and bake them, so in addition to being delicious and comforting, they're also healthy.

Makes about
16 balls

Ready in 1 hour

For the Rice

1 pound Yukon Gold potatoes (about 2 medium), cut into large dice (about 4 cups)

2 cups cooked brown rice (from ⅔ cup uncooked rice)

1 cup tomato sauce or Myrna's Marinara Sauce (page 34; or store-bought oil-free marinara sauce)

¼ cup unsweetened, unflavored plant milk (or water)

¼ cup nutritional yeast (optional)

2 medium garlic cloves, minced (about 1 teaspoon)

Sea salt

Freshly ground black pepper

For the Filling

½ medium yellow onion, cut into ¼-inch dice (about 1 cup)

2 cups cremini mushrooms (or white button mushrooms), trimmed and cut into ¼-inch dice (about 5 ounces)

1 teaspoon minced garlic

½ cup fresh or frozen green peas (about 2½ ounces)

1 tablespoon nutritional yeast (optional)

2 teaspoons finely chopped fresh basil (or 1 teaspoon dried)

1 teaspoon finely chopped fresh thyme (or ½ teaspoon dried)

Sea salt

Pinch of red pepper flakes (optional)

1 cup bread crumbs, plus more for dusting

1 cup Myrna's Marinara Sauce (page 34; or store-bought oil-free marinara sauce)

1. To prepare the rice balls, preheat the oven to 450°F. Line a large baking sheet with parchment paper.

2. Place a steamer basket in a medium saucepan and add 1 to 2 inches of water to the pan. Bring the water to a simmer over medium-high heat. Place the potatoes in

Rustic Pizza Toasts

Makes about
16 to 18 toasts
or about 40
bread sticks

Ready in
45 minutes

These "cheese"-covered toasts are like thick-crust pizza. I cut them into sticks to make an easy-to-eat appetizer. Served whole, the toasts make a comforting lunch or dinner.

1 cup Potato "Cheese" Sauce (page 33)

3 teaspoons finely chopped fresh herbs (any combination of chives,

sage, thyme, marjoram, oregano, and parsley)

1 loaf rustic bread (about 14 ounces), sliced ½-inch thick

1 cup Myrna's Marinara Sauce (page 34; or store-bought oil-free marinara sauce)

1. Preheat the oven to 400°F.

2. Reserve ½ teaspoon of the fresh herbs for garnish. Combine the potato "cheese" sauce with the remaining herbs and stir to combine.

3. Lay the bread slices on two baking sheets and toast for 3 to 4 minutes on each side, until light golden brown. Remove the toast from the oven.

4. Spread a generous layer of the potato "cheese" sauce on each slice and drizzle with marinara sauce.

5. Bake the toasts in the oven for 10 minutes. Remove them from the oven and set aside for a minute or two until they are cool enough to touch. Cut each toast into 1-inch sticks. Garnish with the remaining herbs, and serve right away.

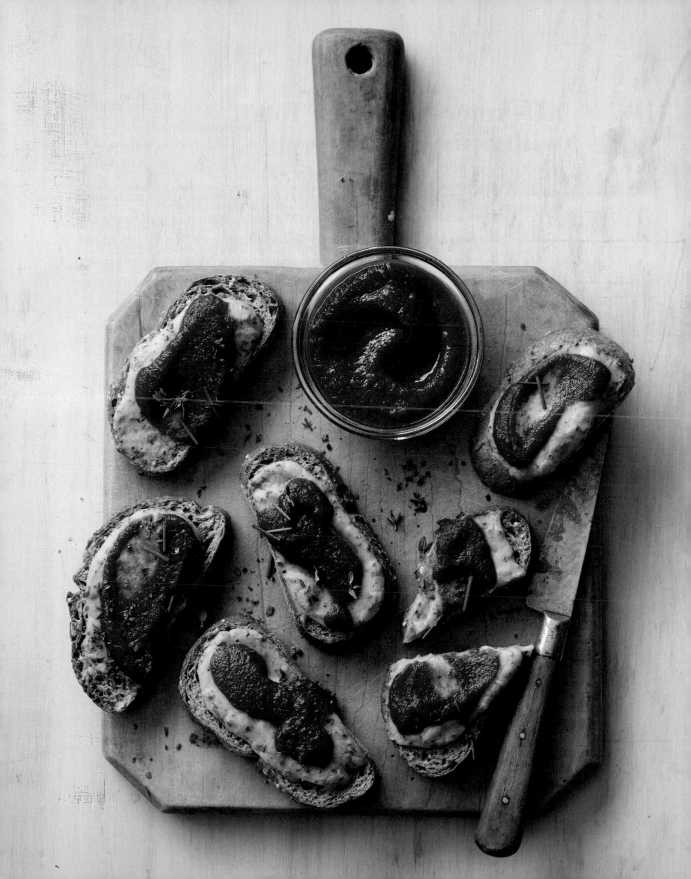

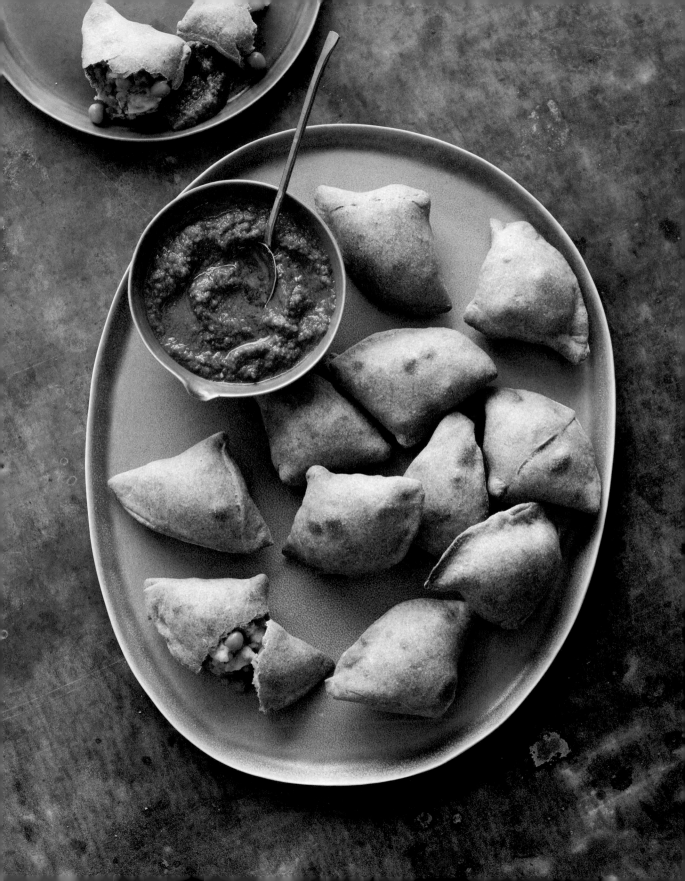

Punjabi Samosas

Samosas are one of the most popular Indian appetizers, both in India and around the world—so much so that I felt an oil-free version was nothing short of a necessity. This recipe is inspired by a version that my sister, Falguni Jalota, makes. She often serves them when she entertains, and I have spent many an hour over the years helping her assemble and fry samosas for her guests. Mine are baked rather than fried, but the flavor and the spirit of them is spot-on.

Makes about 24 samosas

Ready in 1 hour, 30 minutes

For the Filling

1½ pounds russet potatoes (about 3 medium), cut into ½-inch dice

1 cup fresh or frozen green peas (about 5 ounces)

¼ cup finely chopped fresh cilantro

2 tablespoons fresh lemon juice

1 tablespoon plus 1 teaspoon ground coriander

2 teaspoons ground cumin

2 teaspoons grated peeled fresh ginger

½ jalapeño pepper, seeded and minced (optional)

1 teaspoon garam masala

½ teaspoon sea salt

Freshly ground black pepper

For the Crust

1 tablespoon flaxseed meal (brown or golden)

½ cup raw cashews, soaked in hot water for 20 minutes

2 cups whole-wheat flour

½ teaspoon sea salt

Unbleached all-purpose flour (or whole-wheat flour) for dusting

Fresh Cilantro Chutney (page 338) or Nepalese Tomato Chutney (page 339)

1. To prepare the filling, place a steamer basket in a medium saucepan and add 1 to 2 inches of water to the pan. Bring the water to a simmer over medium-high heat. Place the potatoes in the steamer, cover, and steam until tender when pierced with a fork, about 10 minutes. Transfer the potatoes to a large bowl and allow to cool slightly.

2. Mash the potatoes with a potato masher or fork. Add the peas, cilantro, lemon juice, coriander, cumin, ginger, jalapeño, garam masala, and salt and pepper to taste. Mix well.

3. To make the crust, preheat the oven to 425°F. Line two baking sheets with parchment paper.

Lebanese Flatbread with Harissa Hummus and Arugula

Makes 8 pizzas

Ready in
30 minutes

These pita-based flatbreads make great party food. Flatbread is basically a kind of pizza. I call these flatbreads, as opposed to pizza, because they are composed of ingredients including pita bread, hummus, olives, and golden raisins, that are Middle Eastern or North African, not Italian.

"If you're working with dried fruit that is exceptionally hard, soften it by soaking it in water for 10 minutes, or until it is pliable."

8 whole-grain pita breads (see Za'atar Spiced Pita Bread, page 297; or store-bought)

1 medium yellow onion, halved and thinly sliced into half moons (about 2 cups)

Harissa Hummus (page 72)

4 medium tomatoes (about 1½ pounds), sliced ¼-inch thick

8 cups fresh baby arugula, roughly chopped (about 6 ounces)

¼ cup sliced pitted Kalamata olives

¼ cup raisins (or another dried fruit, chopped to the size of raisins)

1. Preheat the oven to 400°F. Line two baking sheets with parchment paper.

2. Spread the pitas in a single layer on the baking sheets and bake for 5 to 7 minutes, until they are golden and lightly crisp, turning them halfway through. Remove from the oven.

3. Sauté the onion in a sauté pan over medium heat for about 10 minutes, until the onion is tender and translucent, stirring frequently to prevent it from sticking to the pan. (Avoid adding water if possible; you want the onion to brown.) Transfer the onion to a plate and set aside.

4. Spread a scant ¼ cup of hummus on each pita. Lay the tomato slices on top and scatter the onion, arugula, olives, and raisins over the tomatoes.

5. Return the pitas to the oven to bake for 10 minutes to warm them through.

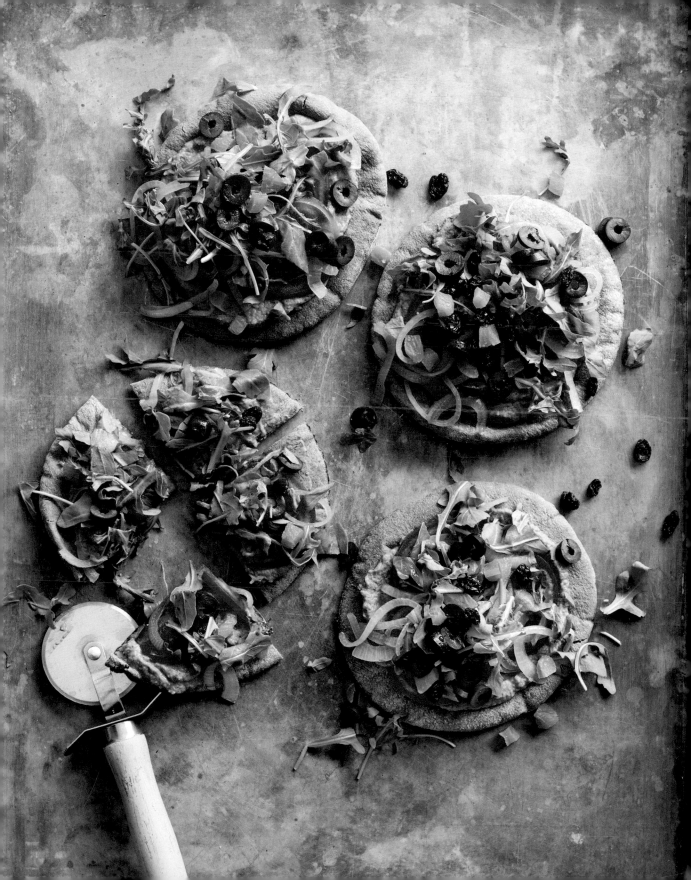

3. Meanwhile, working in batches, put the cabbage, carrot, mushrooms, scallions, and chile into a food processor and pulse to finely chop the vegetables.

4. Transfer the vegetables to a sauté pan and add the tamari, ginger, garlic, turmeric, and lime juice. Stir to combine the ingredients and sauté over medium heat for about 10 minutes, until the liquid released by the vegetables has been cooked off. Add the tofu and cook for about 2 minutes to allow the flavors to meld. Turn off the heat and set aside.

5. Uncover the bowl with the dough and divide the dough into 2-teaspoon-size portions. Roll each portion into a ball. Roll a ball in the cornstarch or arrowroot powder and place it on a cutting board. Using a rolling pin, roll it into a 4-inch disk.

6. Place 1 heaping tablespoon of filling in the center of the disk and gather the edges with your fingers; turn the dough to seal the dumpling closed.

7. Place a steamer basket in a medium saucepan and add 1 to 2 inches of water to the pan. Sprinkle the basket with water and place the finished momo on the steamer basket. Repeat, assembling the remaining momos with the remaining dough and filling.

8. Put the lid on the saucepan and steam the momos for 7 to 10 minutes, until they have puffed up. Use a thin spatula to remove the momos from the steamer basket.

9. Serve hot with chutney on the side for dipping.

TIP: If the momos are sticking to the steamer basket, dip the spatula in water before sliding it under the momos.

STORAGE: Refrigerate in an airtight container up to 3 days. Steam the momos in a steamer for 3–5 minutes until they are warmed through.

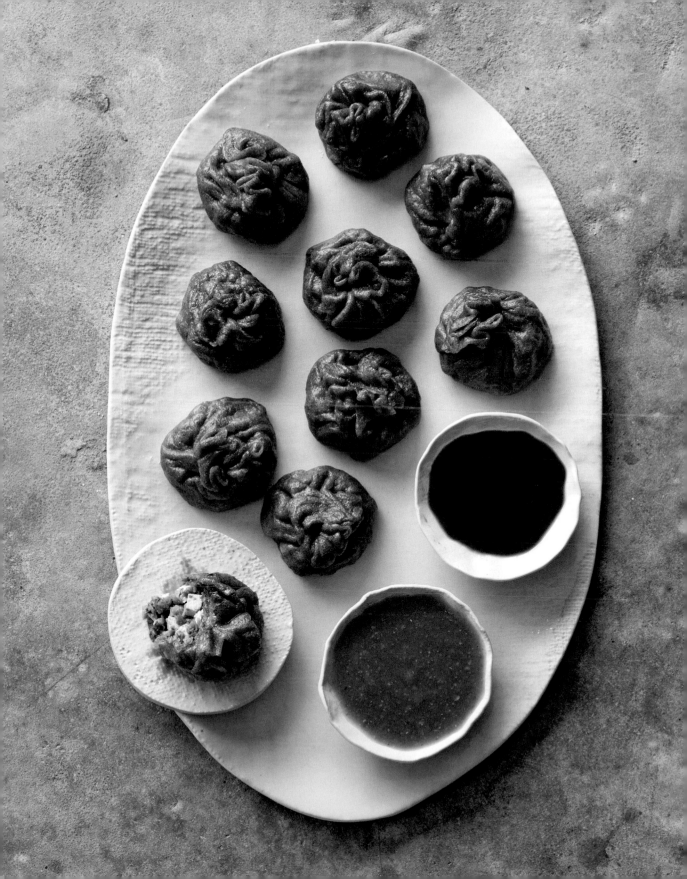

Think about salad and leafy greens come to mind, but it's the little things—chopped vegetables, grains, beans, fruits, nuts, seasonings, and other surprises—that give every salad its unique character. Enjoy these for breakfast, lunch, or dinner.

3 | Salads

Antipasto Salad with Creamy Italian Dressing

Makes about
12 cups

Ready in
20 minutes

This is my version of a classic Italian American antipasto salad with a dressing made from pureed zucchini. Don't feel that you have to follow this recipe exactly; use whatever seasonal vegetables you like in place of those called for here. You can serve the salad drizzled with the dressing or serve the dressing on the side as a dipping sauce.

1 romaine heart, cut into 1-inch pieces (about 4 cups)

1 (15-ounce) can chickpeas, rinsed and drained (about 1½ cups)

6 to 8 small sweet peppers, cut into quarters (about 1½ cups)

1 cup sugar snap peas (about 4 ounces), trimmed and cut in half diagonally

1 cup cherry tomatoes (about 6 ounces), halved

½ head radicchio, thinly sliced

¼ small red onion, thinly sliced (about ¼ cup)

1 small (10- to 15-ounce) jar or can artichoke hearts (packed in water), quartered

¼ cup pitted olives (optional)

6 to 8 pepperoncini, thinly sliced (about ¼ cup)

Creamy Italian Dressing (recipe follows)

1. Pile the lettuce in a large bowl or on a large platter.
2. Arrange the chickpeas, peppers, peas, tomatoes, radicchio, onion, and artichoke hearts over the lettuce in a colorful pattern. Scatter the olives and pepperoncini over the salad. Drizzle with the dressing or serve it as a dipping sauce on the side.

Creamy Italian Dressing

Makes about 1¼ cups

Ready in 10 minutes

I'm always looking for ways to make creamy dressings that are low in fat. In this recipe, I use zucchini, which has a mild flavor and creamy texture, to achieve that. I peel the zucchini to

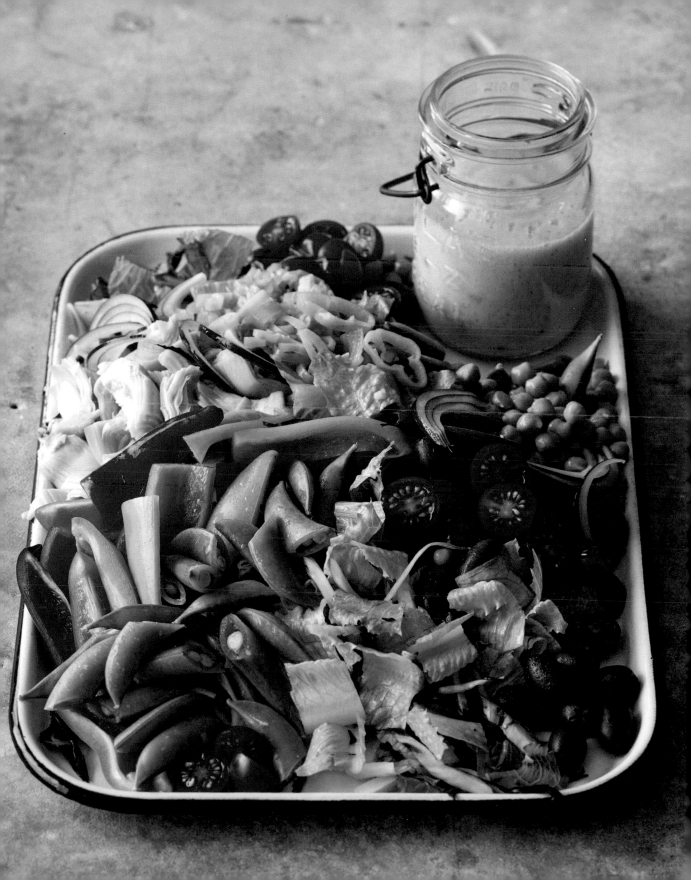

Indonesian Peanut Sauce

Makes about
1¼ cups

Ready in 5 minutes

Indonesian peanut sauce is similar to classic peanut sauce, but it also contains tamarind, which has a sweet, tangy flavor. In addition to being a key component of gado gado, it is delicious as a dip for raw vegetables, or as an alternative wherever Peanut Sauce (page 337) is called for.

⅓ cup peanut butter

2 tablespoons fresh lemon juice

1 tablespoon tamarind paste

1 tablespoon pure maple syrup

1 small garlic clove, roughly chopped

1 small shallot or 1 (1-inch) piece red onion, roughly chopped

1 teaspoon Thai Red Curry Paste (page 251; or ½ teaspoon sambal olek)

Sea salt

Combine all the ingredients in a blender or mini food processor. Add ½ cup water and puree, adding more water if necessary to make a thick, drizzle-able consistency.

STORAGE: Refrigerate in an airtight container for up to 1 week.

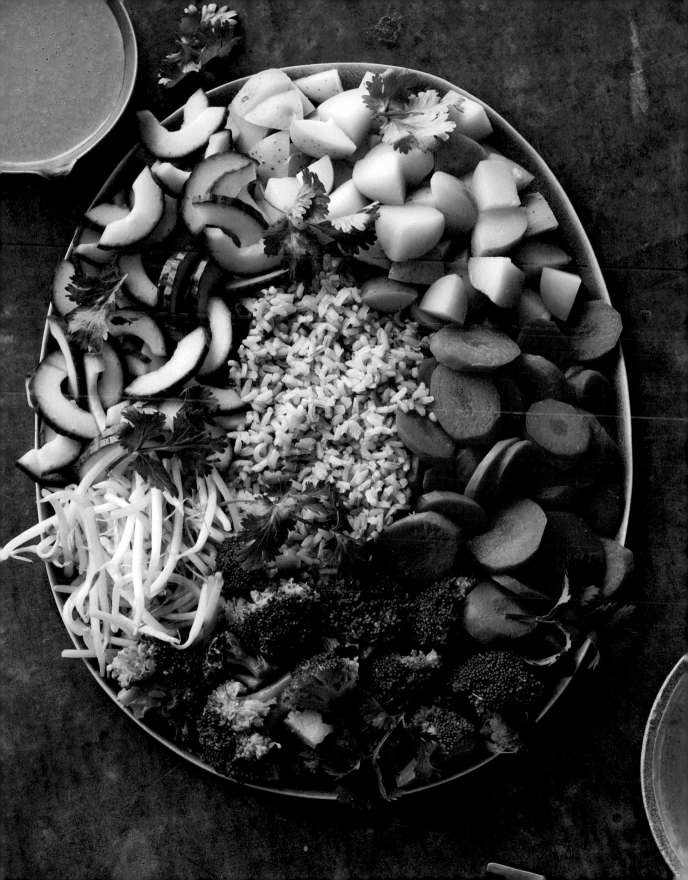

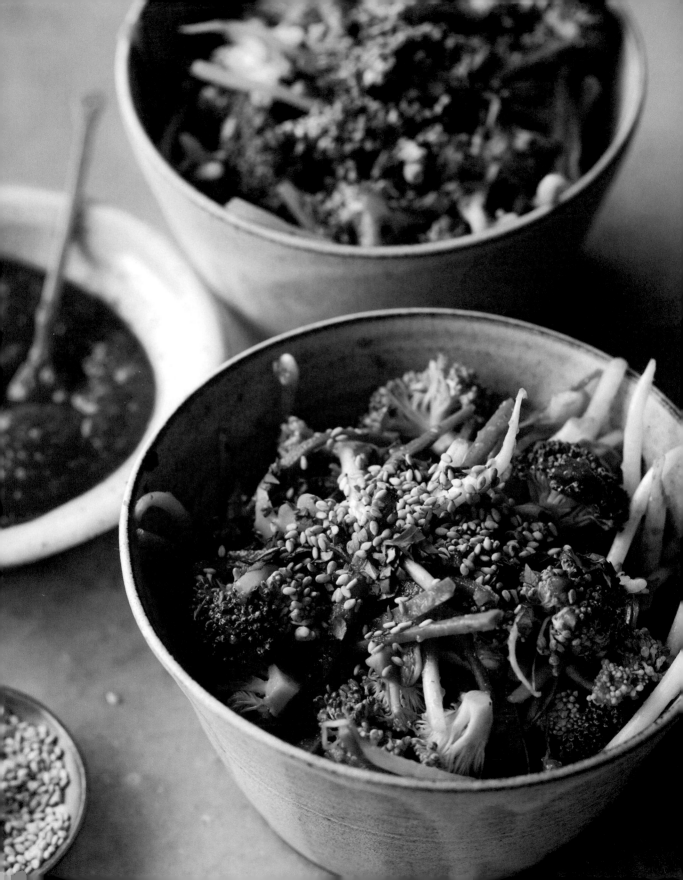

Crunchy Vegetable Salad with Korean Hot Sauce

This mix of crunchy vegetables, including the unusual combination of broccoli and bean sprouts, is brought together by the gochujang, or spicy Korean hot sauce, that the salad is dressed with.

Makes about
4 cups

Ready in
20 minutes

NOTE: Look for Japanese toasted sesame seeds, which come in a tall plastic shaker canister. The canister makes them easy to use and store, and something about the way that they are toasted makes them extremely flavorful. You can find them at gourmet and ethnic markets. I keep a canister of both the black sesame seeds and the white sesame seeds on hand to sprinkle into salads and noodle dishes.

8 ounces broccoli, cut into ½- to ¼-inch florets (about 4 cups)	2 medium carrots, peeled and cut into matchsticks (about 2 cups)	Gochujang (page 343)
4 cups bean sprouts (about 10 ounces)	2 scallions, thinly sliced (white and green parts; about ½ cup)	2 tablespoons finely chopped fresh cilantro
		1 tablespoon toasted sesame seeds

1. Combine the broccoli, bean sprouts, carrots, and scallions in a large bowl.
2. Drizzle the dressing over the mixture and toss to mix the vegetables and coat them with the dressing.
3. Sprinkle the cilantro and sesame seeds over the salad and serve.

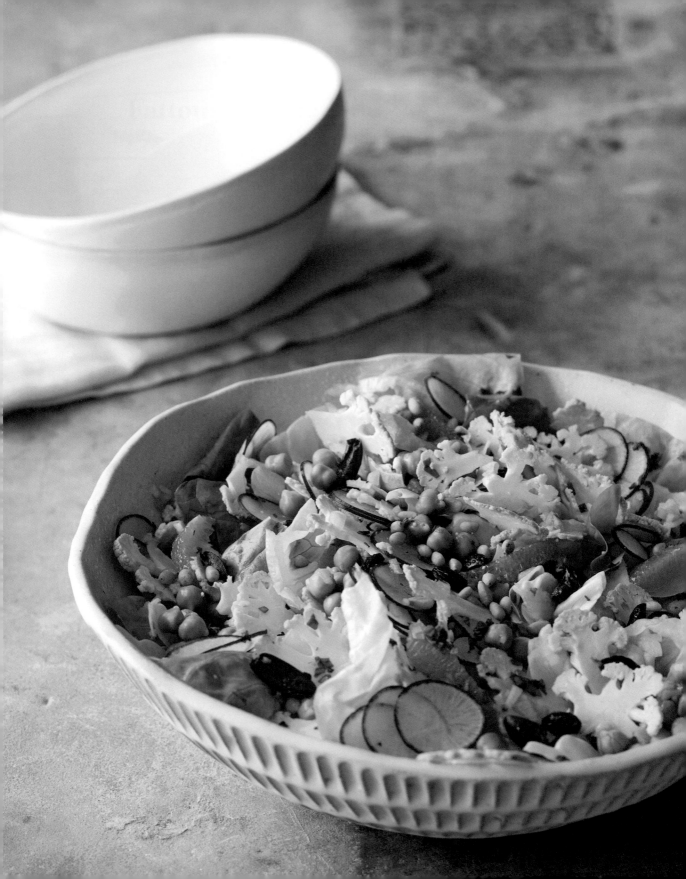

Sicilian Cauliflower and Chickpea Salad

I use a mandoline to shave a whole head of cauliflower into paper-thin slices for this salad, but you can do the same with a large sharp knife. When I can find it, I use Romanesco cauliflower, which has a beautiful bright green shade and unusual cone-shaped florets. To turn this colorful salad into a complete meal, add 1 to 2 cups cooked farro.

Makes about
10 cups

Ready in
25 minutes

For the Dressing

1 medium shallot, finely chopped (about ½ cup)

2 tablespoons white wine vinegar

2 tablespoons fresh lemon juice

1 medium garlic clove, minced (about ½ teaspoon)

Sea salt

Freshly ground black pepper

For the Salad

1 large orange

1 large head Romanesco cauliflower (or another type of cauliflower)

4 cups butter lettuce (about half a head), torn into 1-inch pieces

½ (15-ounce) can chickpeas, rinsed and drained (about ¾ cup)

5 radishes, thinly sliced (about ½ cup)

¼ cup finely chopped fresh basil

2 tablespoons sliced pitted Kalamata olives (optional)

2 tablespoons raisins

2 tablespoons unsalted pine nuts, lightly toasted (optional)

1. To make the dressing, in a small bowl, combine the shallot, vinegar, lemon juice, garlic, and ¼ cup water. Add salt and pepper to taste.

2. To make the salad, peel the orange and break it into segments. Discard the peel.

3. Cut the cauliflower into quarters. Using a mandoline or a large sharp knife, slice the cauliflower into wafer-thin slices and put the slices into a large bowl.

4. Add the lettuce, orange segments, chickpeas, radishes, basil, olives (if you are using them), raisins, and pine nuts (if you are using them) to the bowl. Drizzle the dressing over the salad and toss to combine. Add more salt or pepper to taste. Serve immediately.

STORAGE: Refrigerate in an airtight container for up to 2 days.

Mexican Chopped Salad

Makes about
8 cups

Ready in
30 minutes

In this salad, the vegetables are roasted before being added into the mix. I call for the veggies to be roasted in the oven, but you can also cook them on an outdoor grill. If you want to make the salad more substantial, toss in 2 cups of cooked brown rice, quinoa, or farro or toasted, broken-up corn tortillas.

1 medium zucchini, sliced into ½-inch rounds

1 cup small cherry tomatoes

1 cup fresh or frozen pearl onions, peeled if fresh, cut into quarters

1 medium red, yellow, or orange bell pepper, cored, seeded, and cut into ½-inch strips (about 1 cup)

2 romaine hearts, core removed and discarded, cut into 1-inch pieces (about 8 cups)

1 (15-ounce) can black beans, rinsed and drained (about 1½ cups)

1 cup fresh or frozen corn kernels (from about 1 large cob)

2 tablespoons finely chopped fresh cilantro

2 tablespoons toasted pumpkin seeds

2 tablespoons fresh lime juice

1 teaspoon smoked paprika (or ½ teaspoon ground chipotle)

Sea salt

Four-Chile Salsa (page 342; or store-bought oil-free salsa)

1. Preheat the oven to 500°F. Line a large baking sheet with parchment paper.

2. Spread the zucchini, tomatoes, onions, and bell pepper strips in a single layer on the baking sheet and bake for 15 to 20 minutes, until they are browned in places. Remove the baking sheet from the oven and set aside to cool slightly.

3. Put the lettuce into a large bowl. Add the roasted vegetables, beans, corn, cilantro, pumpkin seeds, lime juice, paprika, and salt to taste and toss gently to combine.

4. Drizzle the salad with salsa and serve.

STORAGE: Refrigerate in an airtight container for up to 2 days.

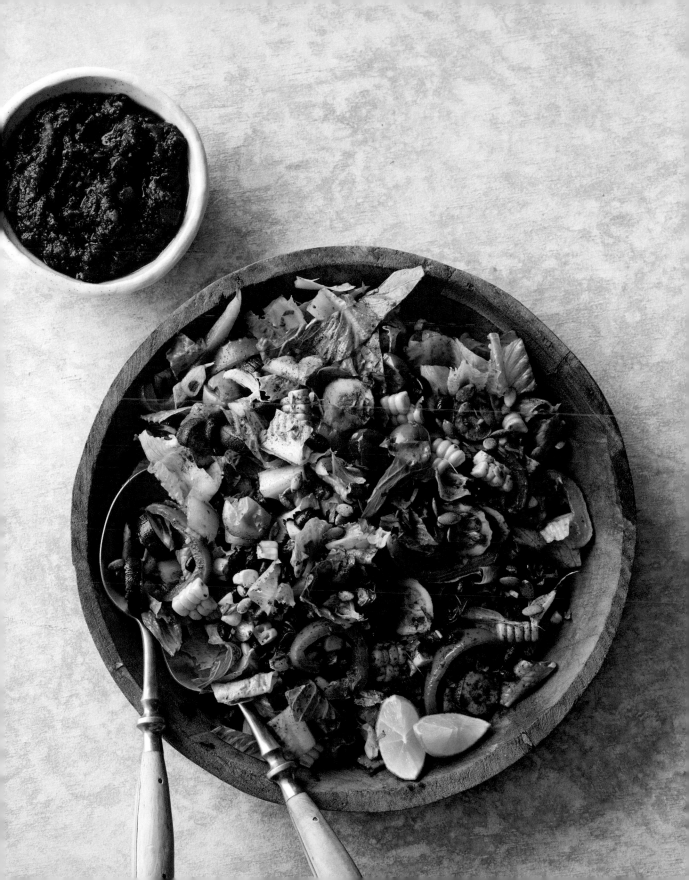

Tunisian Couscous and Carrot Salad

Makes about
10 cups

Ready in
30 minutes

Technically, couscous is a kind of pasta, but it seems so much like a grain in how you cook and eat it that I tend to think of it as a grain. For this salad, you can use fine North African couscous or Israeli couscous, which is larger. The harissa-based dressing tossed into this colorful, hearty salad gives it a bold flair that will delight you and your guests.

1 cup whole-wheat couscous (fine couscous or Israeli couscous)

½ cup Harissa (page 344)

1 bunch kale, stems removed and discarded, leaves shredded (about 4 cups)

1 (15-ounce) can chickpeas, drained and rinsed (about 1½ cups)

2 medium carrots, peeled and grated on the large holes of a box grater (about 1½ cups)

1 medium tomato, cut into ½-inch dice (about 1 cup)

4 scallions, thinly sliced (white and green parts; about 1 cup)

2 tablespoons dried currants

2 tablespoons finely chopped fresh parsley

1. For Israeli couscous, bring 1 cup water to a boil in a medium saucepan over high heat. Reduce the heat to medium-low and simmer, covered, for about 15 minutes, until the liquid is absorbed. For fine couscous, bring 1½ cups water to a boil in a medium saucepan over high heat. Stir in the couscous. Turn off the heat, cover the pot, and let the couscous steep for about 15 minutes, until it is tender. Drain in a colander.

2. Transfer the couscous to a large bowl and fluff it with a fork. Set aside to cool to room temperature.

3. Add the harissa to the bowl with the couscous and toss it gently to distribute the harissa; this also helps prevent the couscous from forming clumps. Add the kale, chickpeas, carrots, tomato, scallions, and currants and toss gently to combine.

4. Garnish with the parsley and serve.

STORAGE: Refrigerate in an airtight container for up to 2 days.

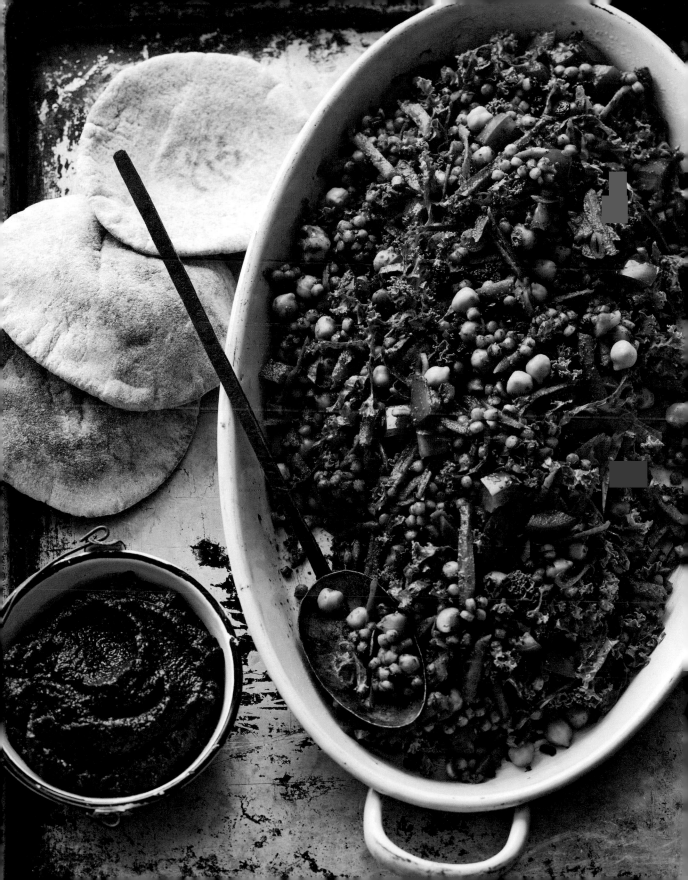

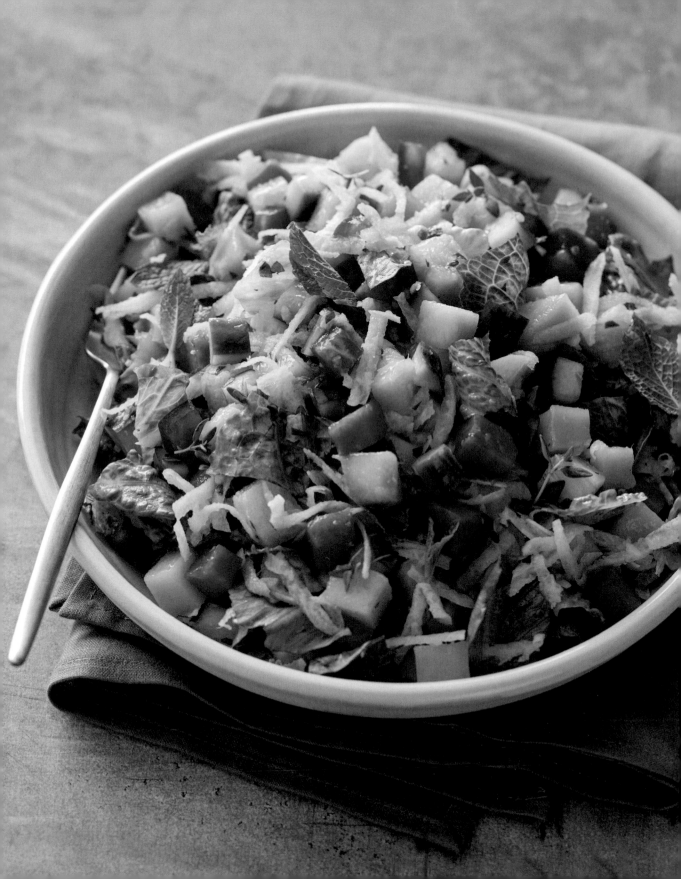

Caribbean Salad with Tropical Fruit

Fruit salad is so often reserved for breakfast, but in this version, I mix the fruit with cucumbers, tomato, lettuce, jicama, and fresh aromatic herbs to turn it into more of a lunchtime meal.

The pineapple, papaya, and mango in this dish are so naturally flavorful and juicy that the salad doesn't need any dressing.

Makes about 8 cups

Ready in 20 minutes

1 romaine heart, core removed and discarded, cut into 1-inch pieces (about 4 cups)

2 medium mangoes, peeled and cut into ½-inch dice (about 2 cups)

1 cup (½-inch-diced) pineapple (about 6 ounces)

6 ounces jicama, peeled and grated on the large holes of a box grater (about 1½ cups)

1 Persian cucumber, cut into ½-inch dice (about 1 cup)

1 medium tomato, cut into ½-inch dice (about 1 cup)

1 cup (½-inch-diced) fresh papaya (or kiwi)

1 tablespoon finely chopped fresh mint

1 tablespoon finely chopped fresh parsley

1 teaspoon finely chopped fresh thyme (optional)

Combine the lettuce, mangoes, pineapple, jicama, cucumber, tomato, and papaya or kiwi in a large mixing bowl. Sprinkle with the mint, parsley, and thyme (if you're using it) and toss to combine the ingredients. Serve right away.

STORAGE: Refrigerate in an airtight container for up to 1 day.

Every culture has its version of grab-and-go foods that are meant to be eaten with your hands. There's something fun and liberating about eating something that doesn't require a fork and knife.

4 | Burgers, Sandwiches, Tacos, and Other Handheld Meals

Huaraches: Mexican Masa "Flatbreads" with Beans and Lime-Spiked Salad

Makes 6 huaraches

Ready in
45 minutes

Huarache, which means "sandal" in Spanish, is a masa cake formed in an oblong shape, like a sandal, which is where this dish gets its name. The cakes are much thicker than tortillas; their texture reminds me of a corn-based pizza crust or flatbread.

These are designed as individual servings, but you can also slice them and serve them as finger food.

For the Beans
1 small yellow onion, cut into ¼-inch dice (about 1 cup)

4 medium garlic cloves, minced (about 2 teaspoons)

2 (15-ounce) cans pinto beans, rinsed and drained (about 3 cups)

2 tablespoons fresh lime juice

Sea salt

For the Huaraches
2 cups corn masa harina

1½ cups thinly sliced romaine lettuce (about half a head)

2 scallions, thinly sliced (white and green parts; about ½ cup)

2 tablespoons fresh lime juice

2 tablespoons finely chopped fresh cilantro

2 avocados, sliced (optional)

Fire-Roasted Tomatillo Salsa (page 336) or Four-Chile Salsa (page 342; or store-bought oil-free salsa)

Chipotle "Sour Cream" (page 335) or Tofu "Sour Cream" (page 334)

1. To make the beans, combine the onion, garlic, and ¼ cup water in a large sauté pan. Cook for about 10 minutes, adding 1 to 2 more tablespoons of water as needed to keep the onion from sticking to the pan, until the onion is tender.

2. Add the beans, lime juice, and 1 cup water and cook for 5 to 7 minutes to allow the flavors to meld. Turn off the heat and mash the beans with a fork or potato masher. Add salt to taste.

3. To make the huaraches, put the masa harina into a medium bowl. Stir in 2 cups water and knead into a smooth dough, adding more water as needed.

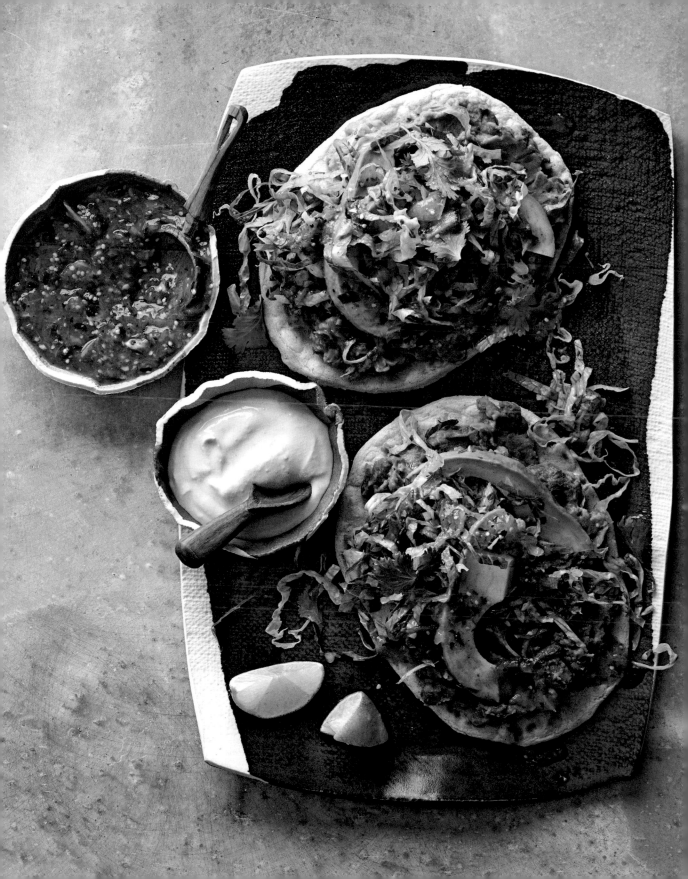

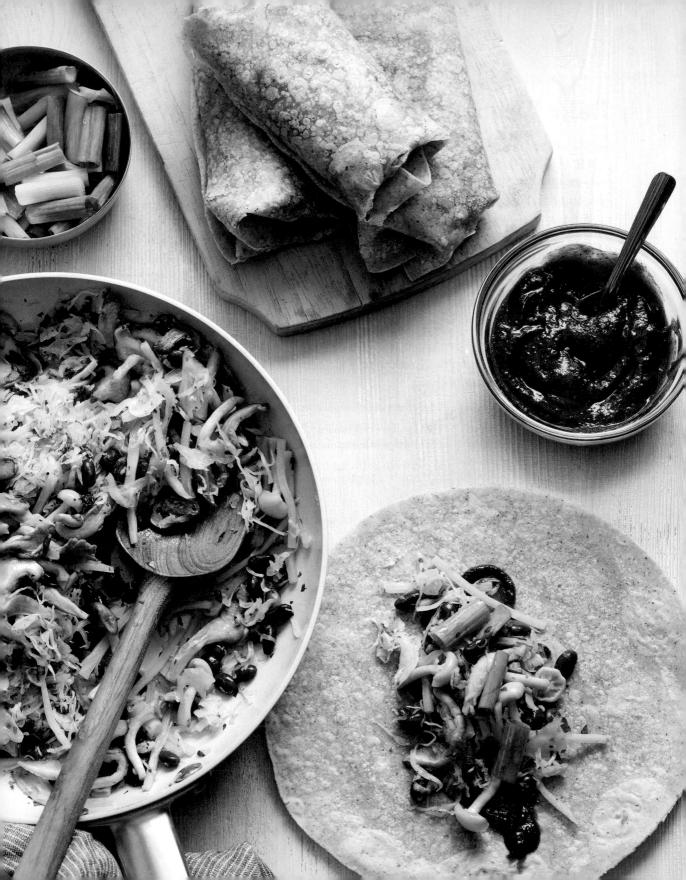

Moo Shu Vegetable Wraps with Hoisin Sauce

Traditionally, Chinese moo shu is a stir-fry and served with hoisin sauce over rice or noodles. However, in Chinese American restaurants, the rice or noodles are replaced with pancakes, which are served separately and used by diners to create their own miniature wraps. In this Chinese American moo shu, I use brown rice tortillas rather than making my own pancakes.

Makes 4 wraps

Ready in
25 minutes

6 cups assorted wild mushrooms, trimmed and thinly sliced (about 5 ounces)

4 medium garlic cloves, minced (about 2 teaspoons)

1 (15-ounce) can black soybeans or black beans,

rinsed and drained (about 1½ cups)

4 cups shredded green cabbage (about 10 ounces)

8 ounces bamboo shoots, cut into julienne (thinly sliced)

4 scallions, cut into 1-inch lengths (white and green parts; about 1 cup)

¼ cup finely chopped fresh cilantro

4 brown rice tortillas (or whole-wheat tortillas)

Hoisin Sauce (recipe follows, or store-bought)

1. Combine the mushrooms and garlic in a large sauté pan (or wok) over medium-high heat and sauté for about 5 minutes, until the mushrooms are tender. Increase the heat to high. Add the beans, cabbage, and bamboo shoots and half the scallions and cook for 3 to 5 minutes, until the cabbage is just wilted. Turn off the heat and stir in the cilantro.

2. One at a time, heat the tortillas in a sauté pan over medium heat until they are warm and pliable. Wrap them in a kitchen towel to keep them soft and warm.

3. To assemble the wraps, spread the hoisin sauce in a thick stripe down the center of each tortilla. Spoon the filling over the sauce, dividing it evenly, and scatter the rest of the scallions on top. Fold the ends up and the sides inward to create a wrap. Serve with the remaining hoisin sauce on the side.

STORAGE: Refrigerate in an airtight container, wrapped in wax paper, for up to 2 days. Remove wax paper before reheating in a skillet or toaster oven until warmed through.

7 minutes for the underside to brown. Remove the pupusa from the griddle to a platter. Continue forming pupusas and adding them to the griddle or sauté pan as they are ready.

6. To serve, top with salsa and *curtido*.

STORAGE: Refrigerate in an airtight container for up to 3 days; heat them in a preheated 350°F oven until they are warmed through.

Red Cabbage Slaw

Makes about
3 cups

Ready in 30
minutes

The traditional name for this slaw is *curtido*. It is a quick-pickled slaw that is piled onto pupusas. I like to make a big batch of this to keep in the refrigerator. In addition to using it on the Spinach and "Cheese" Pupusas, I pile it into tacos and sandwiches, onto tostadas, and anywhere else I think that its color and crunch would be welcome.

2 cups shredded red
cabbage

1 small carrot, peeled and
grated (about ½ cup)

1 small yellow onion, thinly
sliced (about 1 cup)

¼ cup white wine vinegar

¼ cup fresh lime juice

Sea salt

Combine the cabbage, carrot, onion, vinegar, lime juice, salt to taste, and ¼ cup water in a large bowl. Set aside for at least 30 minutes to pickle the vegetables.

STORAGE: Refrigerate in an airtight container for up to 3 days.

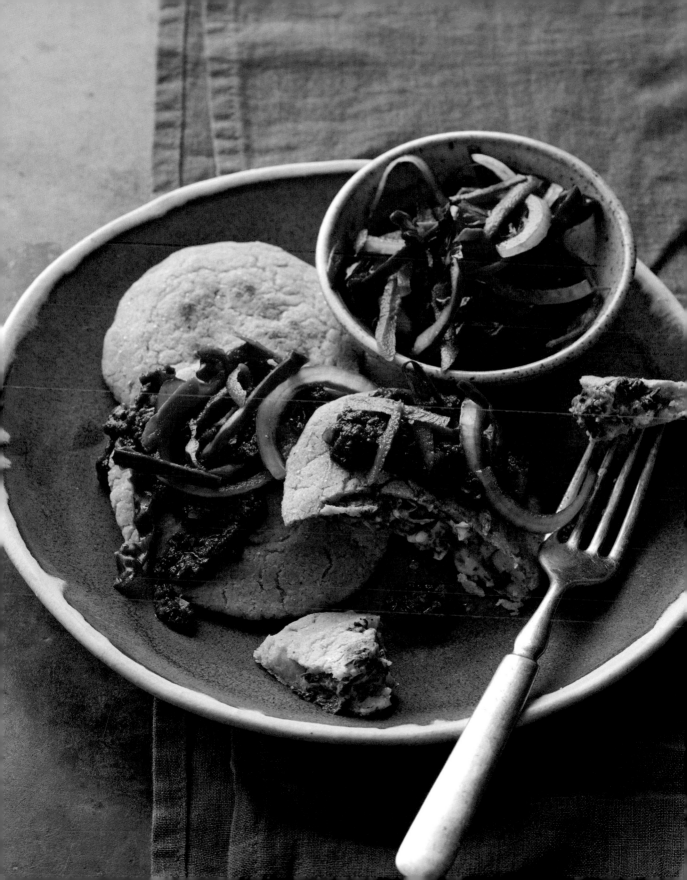

lemon juice, and salt and pepper to taste. Cook, uncovered, until the water is absorbed, about 10 minutes.

3. Heat the tortillas in a sauté pan over medium heat until pliable, about 20 seconds on each side. Cover with a damp cloth to keep them warm and soft until serving.

4. To assemble the wraps, heap a small handful (about ¼ cup) of spinach leaves onto the middle of one tortilla. Top with ¾ cup of the filling and spoon 1 tablespoon of chutney over the filling. Fold the sides of tortilla over the filling, then roll up to close the wrap. Repeat, assembling the remaining wraps with the remaining tortillas and filling.

5. Serve the wraps with the remaining chutney on the side.

STORAGE: Refrigerate for up to 3 days, wrapped in wax paper. Remove wax paper before reheating until they are warmed through.

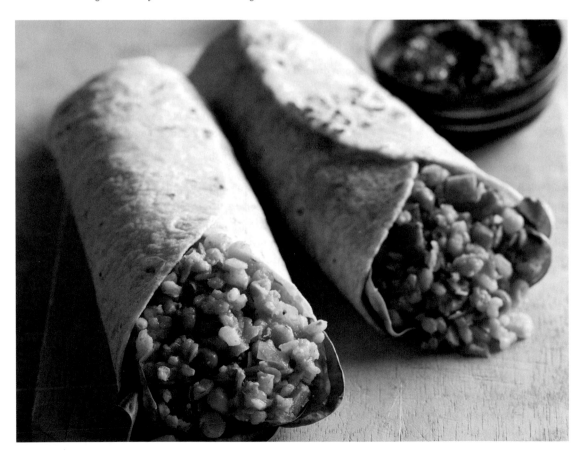

Polenta Pizza with Summer Garden Vegetables

I love the corn flavor and creamy texture of polenta, and I love pizza—so naturally I wanted to create a polenta pizza. I use a summery mix of vegetables to top this pizza; use any combination of vegetables you like or that is in season. The Cashew Chickpea "Cheese" is a wonderful part of this dish; if you don't have the time to make it, sprinkle nutritional yeast on the pizza instead.

Makes 8 4-by-5-inch slices

Ready in 1 hour

For the Crust
2 cups polenta

1 tablespoon flaxseed meal (preferably golden)

For the Topping
3 medium zucchini, thinly sliced (about 4½ cups)

2 cups mushrooms, trimmed and thinly sliced (about 5 ounces)

2 medium red bell peppers, cored, seeded, and thinly sliced (about 2 cups)

1 medium red onion, thinly sliced (about 2 cups)

1½ cups Myrna's Marinara Sauce (page 34; or store-bought oil-free marinara sauce)

3 tablespoons tomato paste

Frozen Cashew Chickpea "Cheese" (page 35) or nutritional yeast

Sea salt

8 to 10 fresh basil leaves, torn into pieces

1. Line 2 large baking sheets with parchment paper.

2. Mix the polenta and flaxseed together in a small bowl. Bring 5½ cups water to a boil in a large saucepan over high heat. Add the polenta-flax mixture in a slow and steady stream, whisking constantly to break up any clumps. Reduce the heat to low and simmer, stirring occasionally, until the water is absorbed and the polenta is cooked, 7 to 10 minutes. The polenta should be a thick batterlike consistency, but it shouldn't be so thick that you can't move the whisk through it. If it is too thin, cook it a while longer. If it is too thick, add a bit more water.

3. Dump the polenta onto one of the baking sheets and use a wet rubber spatula to spread it into a rectangle ½ inch thick. Wet the spatula again and use it to pat the

edges of the polenta to create a clean, straight edge. Set aside to cool to room temperature. When it has cooled, use a long, serrated knife to cut the sheet of polenta into eight equal-sized rectangles (about 4½ by 5 inches).

4. Preheat the oven to 400°F.

5. Combine the zucchini, mushrooms, bell peppers, and onion in a sauté pan and cook over medium heat for 5 to 7 minutes, until the vegetables are tender, adding as little water as possible to the pan to prevent them from sticking. (You don't want the vegetables to be wet when you put them on the pizza.) Turn off the heat.

6. Use a metal spatula to carefully move half of the sliced polenta rectangles onto the second baking sheet.

7. Stir the marinara sauce and tomato paste together in a small bowl. Spread a generous layer of the sauce (2 to 3 tablespoons) onto each rectangle and top with the sautéed vegetables. Grate the "cheese" liberally or sprinkle nutritional yeast over each slice.

8. Place the pizzas in the oven to bake for about 20 minutes, until crispy and golden brown. Remove the pizzas from the oven. Sprinkle with salt and garnish with the basil. Serve hot.

STORAGE: Refrigerate in an airtight container for up to 3 days; heat them in a preheated 350°F oven for 20 minutes until they are warmed through.

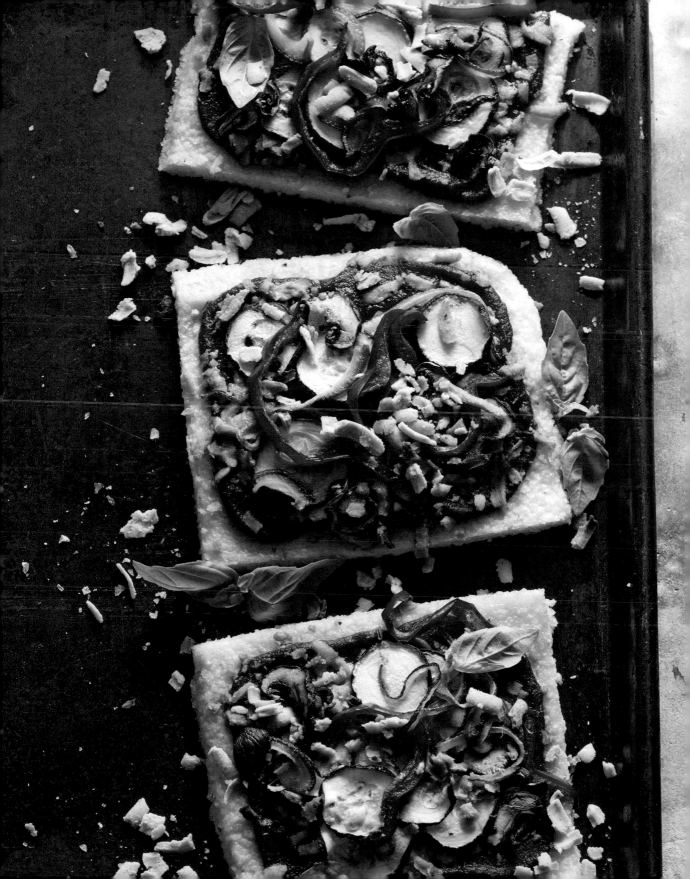

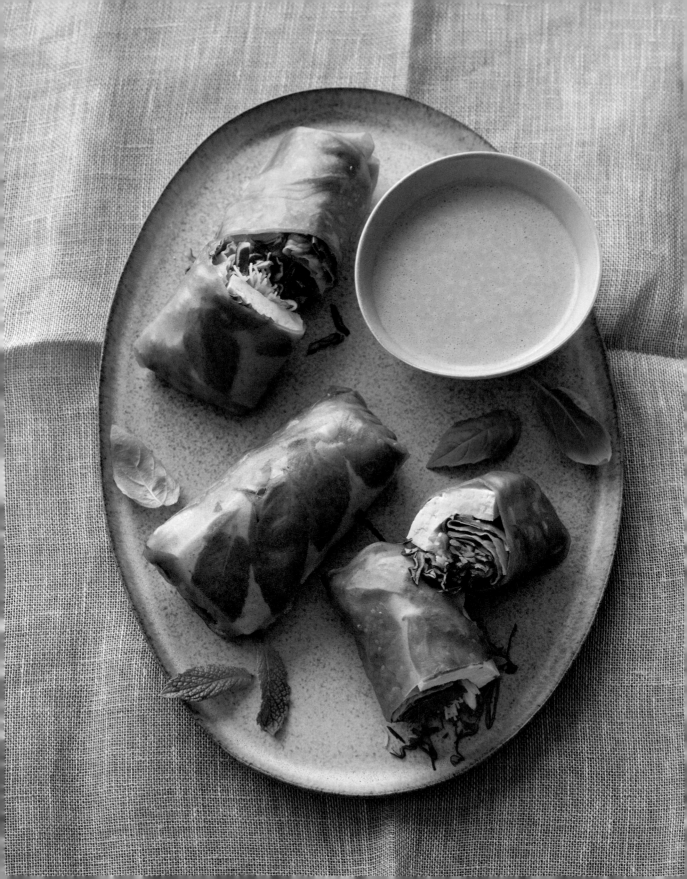

Vietnamese Summer Rolls

Summer rolls are one of my go-to restaurant and takeout foods. One of our top spots in LA for them is the vegan Vietnamese restaurant called Vinh Loi Tofu. The owner, Kevin Tran, and Brian are old friends; Brian has been going to his restaurant for many years. When I started going there with Brian, I was naturally curious and asked Kevin about making summer rolls. He was very generous about answering my questions and gave me a basic tutorial. One thing Kevin taught me about making the rolls is to layer two sheets for each roll, which makes the wrap stronger so it doesn't tear when you roll it. He also taught me to use fillings that are pliable, such as grated vegetables and lettuce with the stems removed. With those tips in mind, I came up with this recipe.

Makes 10 rolls

Ready in
45 minutes

1 (12- to 16-ounce) package extra-firm tofu, drained

2 ounces Thai-style brown rice noodles (or any whole-grain noodles, such as soba or udon noodles or whole-grain pasta)

20 (8½-inch) rice paper sheets

20 large romaine lettuce leaves (about 2 heads), rinsed and dried thoroughly

2 medium carrots, peeled and grated on the large holes of a box grater (about 1½ cups)

1 cup shredded red cabbage

40 Thai basil leaves (or regular basil leaves)

40 fresh mint leaves

1 scallion, thinly sliced diagonally (white and green parts; about 2 tablespoons)

Peanut Sauce (page 337) or Hoisin Sauce (page 140; or store-bought)

1. Bring a medium saucepan of water to a boil over high heat. Add the tofu. Reduce the heat to medium and simmer the tofu for 2 minutes. Remove to a bed of paper towels and pat dry. Slice the tofu ⅓ inch thick and set aside to cool to room temperature.

2. Cook the noodles according to the package instructions. Drain in a colander and run cold water over them to stop them from cooking. Using scissors, snip the noodles into 2- to 3-inch-long pieces. Set aside.

4. Transfer the burger mixture to a food processor. Add the parsley, nutritional yeast, tomato paste, vinegar, kasha, and salt and pepper to taste and pulse until the mixture is coarsely chopped.

5. Turn the burger mixture into a medium bowl. Scoop up a heaping ½ cup of the burger mixture and form it into a 1-inch-thick patty. Place the patty on the prepared baking sheet and repeat with the rest of the mixture.

6. Place the baking sheet with the patties in the oven and bake for 25 minutes. Remove from the oven and flip each patty over using a thin spatula. (If the patties stick to the sheet, let them cool for 5 minutes and then flip them.) Return the patties to the oven to bake for another 25 minutes.

7. Serve the patties on toasted burger buns. Top with dill slaw and serve with ketchup and mustard on the side.

STORAGE: Refrigerate in an airtight container for up to 3 days; heat them in a preheated 350°F oven for 20 minutes until they are warmed through.

Dill Slaw

Makes about 3 cups

Ready in 5 minutes

This simple slaw adds flavor and crunch to just about any sandwich.

⅓ cup almond flour

2 tablespoons fresh lemon juice

1 tablespoon ground chia seeds (or brown or golden flaxseed meal)

1 tablespoon white wine vinegar

½ tablespoon Dijon mustard

Sea salt

Freshly ground black pepper

3 cups shredded green cabbage (about 8 ounces or ¼ small cabbage)

¼ cup finely chopped fresh dill

1. Combine the almond flour, lemon juice, chia seeds, vinegar, mustard, and salt and pepper to taste in a large bowl. Add the cabbage and massage the dressing into it to help it break down. Set aside for 10 minutes.

2. Just before serving, add the dill and toss to combine.

STORAGE: Refrigerate in an airtight container for up to 3 days.

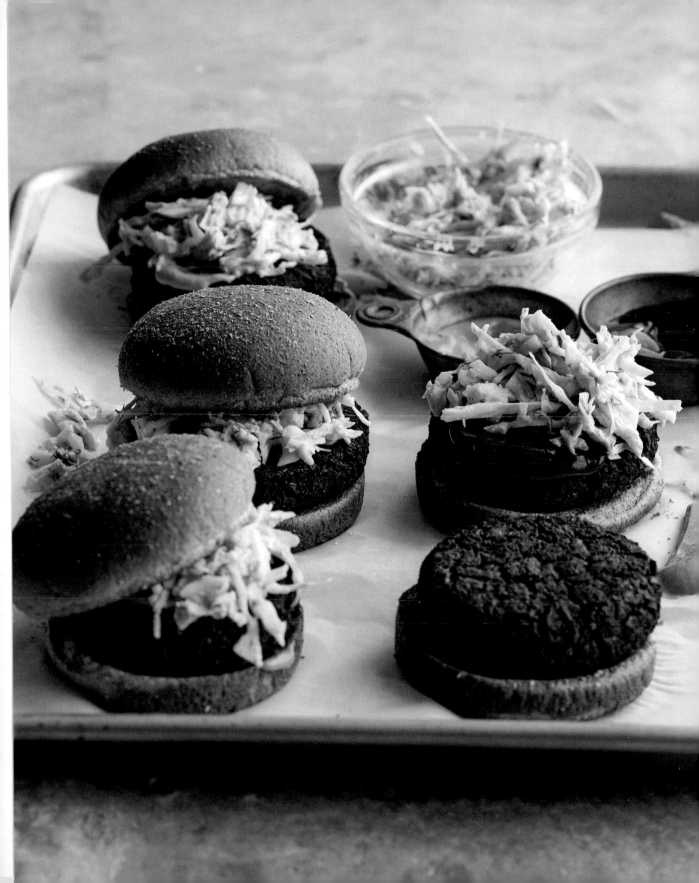

Prepared in a myriad of ways, vegetable side dishes make the perfect partner to soups, salads, and baked dishes. These delicious offerings from around the world will contribute one more element to a spread, turning a meal into a feast.

5 | Warm Veggie Sides

Baked Whole Cauliflower with Red Pepper Romesco and Pesto Bread Crumbs

Makes 1 head of cauliflower

Ready in 45 minutes

One day I was visiting my aunt Malti Thacker, who was making lunch for our family. I was just a child sitting at the dinner table, when out of the oven came a baked, whole cauliflower, covered with a delicious tomato sauce and seasoned with wonderful herbs and spices. I still remember the distinctive taste and lovely presentation. Only for this book, many years later, did I dare go where my aunt and few others have gone: to turn a whole head of cauliflower into a delightful side dish.

1 medium head cauliflower (about 2 pounds)

1 cup Red Pepper Romesco (recipe follows)

Pesto Bread Crumbs (recipe follows)

1. Preheat the oven to 350°F. Line a baking sheet with parchment paper.

2. Rinse the cauliflower and remove the leaves at the base, keeping the stem intact.

3. Place the cauliflower base side down in a medium saucepan. Add enough water to come to the bottom of the head but not so much that the florets are submerged in water. Cover the pot and bring the water to a boil over high heat. Reduce the heat to medium-low and steam the cauliflower until it is tender when pierced with a fork, about 10 minutes. Turn off the heat and uncover the pan. Use tongs to remove the cauliflower from the pan and put it on the baking sheet to cool.

4. Using a spoon or spatula, coat the surface of the cauliflower with the red pepper sauce; it will be a thick coat. Sprinkle the bread crumbs over the cauliflower and bake it in the oven for about 20 minutes, until the bread crumbs are golden brown and crispy.

STORAGE: The cauliflower will keep, refrigerated in a covered container, for up to 4 days. Heat in a 350°F oven until warmed through.

Red Pepper Romesco

Traditional romesco is a condiment from Spain made with dry chiles, nuts, and oil. In this recipe, I make the sauce from sweet roasted red peppers and spicy ground chiles. I use a combination of ground New Mexican chile powder for its bright flavor, and ancho chile powder for its smokiness; use whatever chile powder you like or have. In addition to coating the whole head of cauliflower in the recipe for Baked Whole Cauliflower with Red Pepper Romesco and Pesto Bread Crumbs (recipe on page 160), this sauce makes a delicious dipping sauce for raw or steamed veggies.

Makes about
2 cups

Ready in
20 minutes

6 ounces jarred roasted red bell peppers (about 1 cup)

2 medium carrots (about 6 ounces), sliced ½ inch thick

1 medium shallot (about 1 ounce), peeled and cut into quarters

3 medium garlic cloves, minced (about ½ tablespoon)

1 tablespoon tomato paste

½ tablespoon New Mexico chile powder (or to taste)

½ tablespoon ancho chile powder (or to taste)

1 teaspoon dried oregano

Pinch of cayenne pepper

1 teaspoon arrowroot powder

1 tablespoon fresh lemon juice

Sea salt

Freshly ground black pepper

1. Combine the bell pepper, carrots, shallot, garlic, tomato paste, New Mexico chile powder, ancho chile powder, oregano, and cayenne pepper in a medium saucepan. Add ½ cup water and bring to a boil over high heat. Reduce the heat to medium-low and simmer for about 10 minutes, until the carrots are tender.

2. Combine the arrowroot with 1 tablespoon water in a small bowl and mix with a fork until no lumps remain. (This mixture is called a slurry.) Stir the slurry into the pan with the vegetables and cook for about 1 minute, until the sauce starts to thicken. Turn off the heat and set aside to cool slightly.

3. Transfer the vegetables and liquid to a blender or food processor. Add the lemon juice and blend into a paste, adding 1 to 2 tablespoons of water if needed to get the blender moving. Add salt and pepper to taste.

STORAGE: Refrigerate the sauce in a container with a tight-fitting lid for up to 1 week or freeze for up to 1 month.

Pesto Bread Crumbs

Makes about 1 cup

Ready in 5 minutes

Sprinkle these herby bread crumbs over pasta, pizza, or vegetables and even over salads. In the summertime, when basil is sold in enormous bunches, I like to double the recipe so I have the bread crumbs on hand in the days and weeks ahead.

1 cup packed fresh basil

⅓ cup bread crumbs

⅓ cup nutritional yeast

2 tablespoons fresh lemon juice

1 medium garlic clove

Sea salt (optional)

Freshly ground black pepper

Place the basil, bread crumbs, nutritional yeast, lemon juice, and garlic in a food processor and pulse until the ingredients form a coarse crumble. Add salt (if you're using it) and pepper to taste. If the bread crumbs form lumps after blending them, spread them out on a baking sheet and set them aside for about 20 minutes to dry out.

STORAGE: Store the bread crumbs in an airtight container at room temperature for up to 4 days.

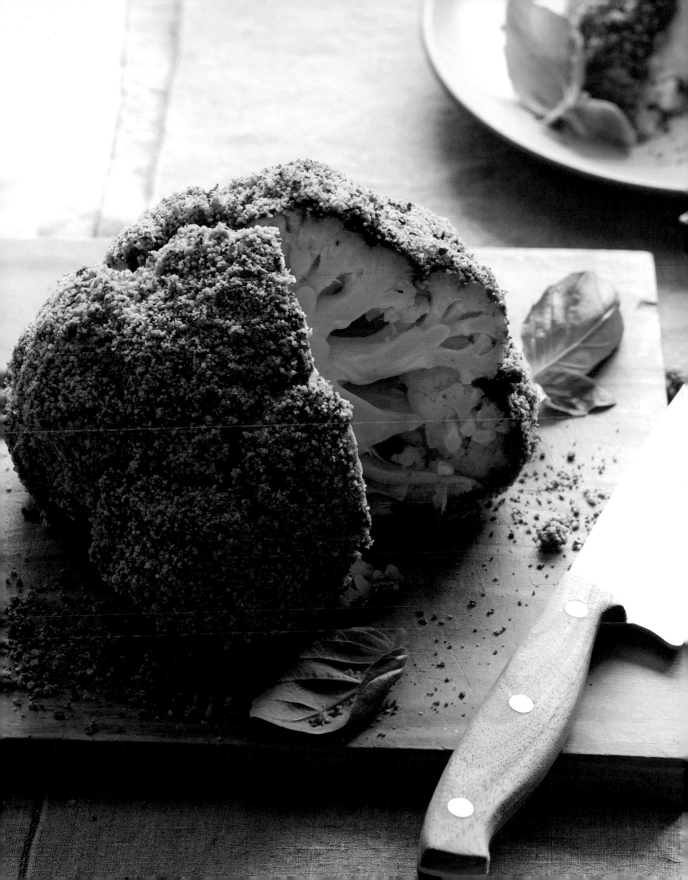

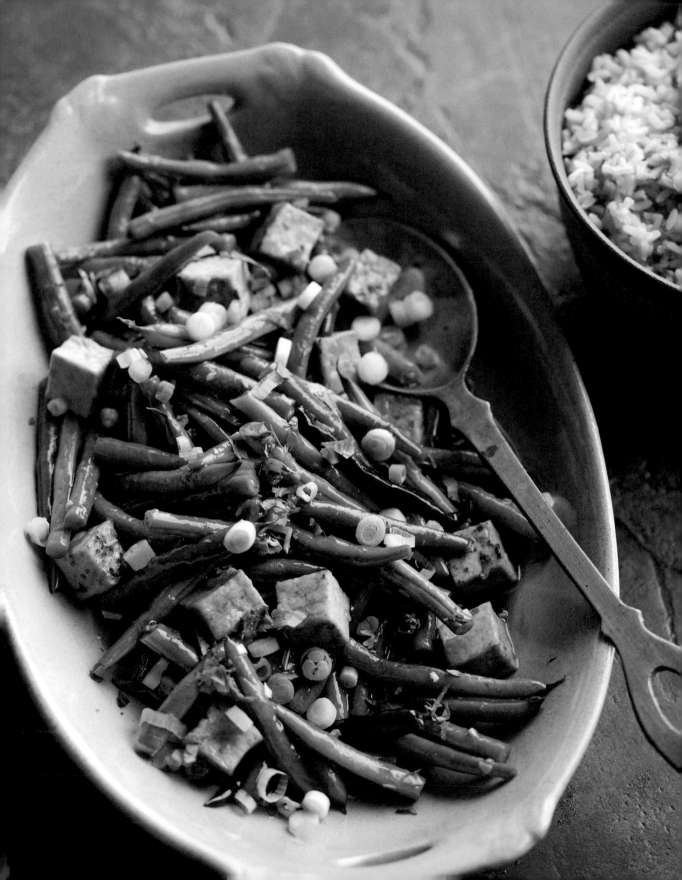

Manchurian Green Beans with Tofu

Among the various cuisines you will find in India is Indo-Chinese food. A small group of Chinese immigrants settled in east India around the eighteenth century, introducing Chinese cuisine to the local population. Over the years, the popularity of this food spread all over country, adapting to Indian taste preferences along the way. The Manchurian sauce that provides flavor for this dish is one of the popular sauces used in Indo-Chinese cuisine.

Makes about 6 cups

Ready in 30 minutes

For the Green Beans
½ (12- to 16-ounce) package extra-firm tofu

1½ pounds green beans, ends trimmed, cut into 3-inch pieces

2 scallions, thinly sliced (white and green parts; about ½ cup)

2 tablespoons finely chopped fresh cilantro

For the Sauce
2 medium garlic cloves, minced (about 1 teaspoon)

1 (2-inch) piece finely chopped, peeled fresh ginger (about 3 tablespoons)

2 árbol chiles (or other small dried red chiles, such as Thai or Indian red chiles)

¼ cup low-sodium tamari (or low-sodium soy sauce)

2 tablespoons fresh lemon juice

2 tablespoons arrowroot powder

1. Drain the tofu and press it between your hands to remove excess liquid. Cut the tofu into 1-inch cubes. Place the cubes in a large nonstick sauté pan over medium heat and cook for about 5 minutes, until golden and crispy on all sides.

2. Meanwhile, to make the sauce, in a separate, large nonstick sauté pan, combine the garlic, ginger, and chiles and toast over medium heat for about 2 minutes, until they are aromatic, stirring constantly so they don't burn. Add the green beans and ¾ cup water. Increase the heat to high and bring to a boil. Reduce the heat to medium and simmer for 5 to 7 minutes, until the beans are cooked but still crunchy. (Cook them for about 3 minutes if you like your vegetables al dente.)

3. Combine the soy sauce, lemon juice, arrowroot, and ¼ cup water to make a slurry and whisk with a fork until no lumps remain. Pour the slurry into the sauté pan and cook, stirring constantly, until the sauce thickens, about 3 minutes. Add the tofu and cook for 5 to 7 minutes, until the sauce coats the tofu and beans. Stir in the scallions and cilantro. Serve warm.

STORAGE: Refrigerate in an airtight container for up to 1 week.

Baked Brussels Sprouts in Creamy Mustard Dressing

Makes about
4 cups

Ready in
30 minutes

Brussels sprouts, when prepared well, are transformed from a not-very-popular vegetable into something really delicious. In this recipe, I shave the Brussels sprouts and then bake them in a creamy mustard sauce; the slight sweetness of the sauce complements the natural bitterness of the vegetable. I like to shred my own Brussels sprouts, since I find that the pre-shredded ones in the grocery store are dried out. For the shredding, you can use a knife, but a food processor or mandoline would make the task easier.

1 pound Brussels sprouts, sliced ⅛- to ¼-inch thick (about 6 cups)

1 cup fresh or frozen green peas (about 5 ounces)

¼ cup almond flour

1 tablespoon Dijon mustard

½ tablespoon low-sodium tamari (or low-sodium soy sauce)

2 tablespoons white wine vinegar

Freshly ground black pepper

1. Preheat the oven to 350°F.

2. Spread the Brussels sprouts on a baking sheet. Drizzle with ½ cup water and bake in the oven for 10 minutes to soften. Remove the baking sheet from the oven.

3. Increase the oven temperature to 425°F.

4. Stir the peas in with the Brussels sprouts and return the baking sheet to the oven. Cook until the Brussels sprouts begin to brown around the edges, 10 to 15 minutes.

5. Meanwhile, combine the almond flour, mustard, tamari, and vinegar in a blender. Add ¼ cup water and blend until smooth. Add pepper to taste.

6. Remove the baking sheet from the oven and drizzle ¼ cup of the dressing over the vegetables. Toss to coat the vegetables with the dressing. Add more as desired, and serve the remaining dressing on the side.

7. Serve warm or chilled.

STORAGE: Refrigerate the cooked vegetables for up to 4 days. Transfer the remaining dressing to a jar with a tight-fitting lid and refrigerate for up to 1 week.

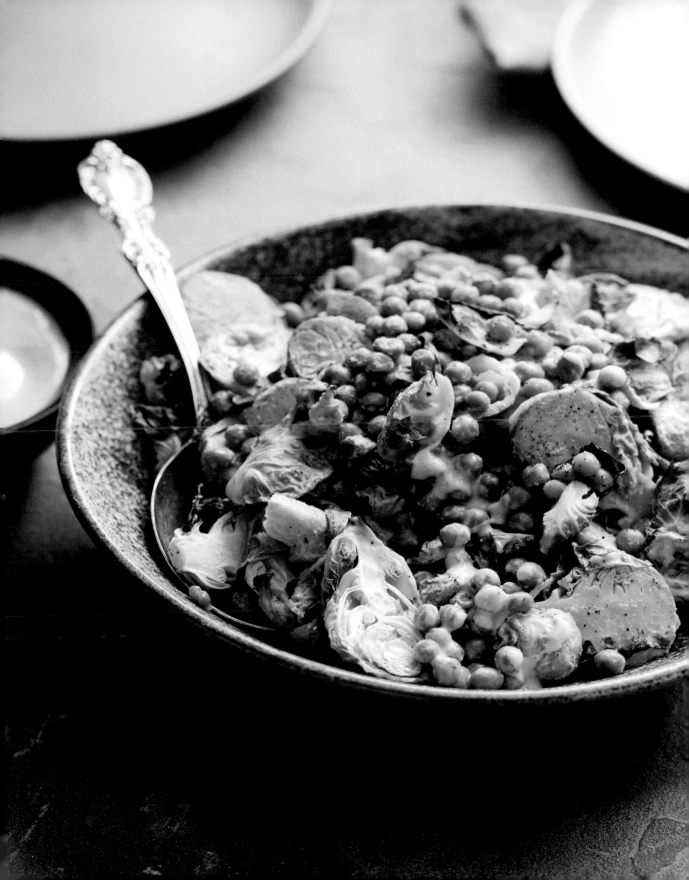

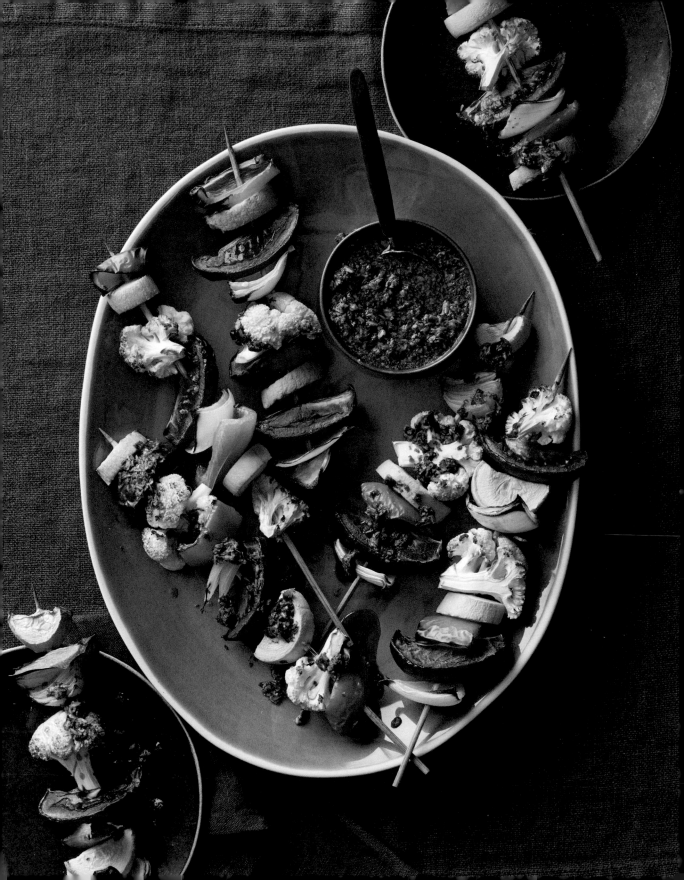

Summer Vegetable Skewers with Chimichurri

The vegetables for these skewers are cooked in the oven, but you can also cook them on an outdoor grill. They make a perfect vegetable side for a backyard barbecue. Chimichurri, an Argentine condiment made of fresh parsley and cilantro, is drizzled on the skewers when they are ready to serve, giving them a bright, herby flavor that is the essence of summer.

Makes 10 to 12 skewers or about 6 cups

Ready in 40 minutes

NOTE: To cook these on a backyard grill, cook them over medium-high heat; the cooking times will be the same.

10 to 12 bamboo or metal skewers

1 red, yellow, or orange bell pepper, cored, seeded, and cut into 2-inch pieces

1 medium summer squash, cut into ½-inch half moons

½ medium yellow onion, cut into 2-inch pieces

1 cup cauliflower florets (about 4 ounces)

2 Roma tomatoes, each cut into 6 wedges

Chimichurri (page 340)

Sea salt

1. Preheat the oven to 425°F. Line a baking sheet with parchment paper. Soak the bamboo skewers in hot water for 15 minutes.

2. Put the vegetable pieces alternately on the skewers and lay the skewers on the prepared baking sheet. Bake for 30 to 40 minutes, until golden brown around the edges.

3. Remove from the oven, drizzle liberally with the sauce, and sprinkle with salt. Place the skewers on a serving platter and serve with the remaining sauce in a dipping bowl.

STORAGE: Refrigerate in an airtight container for up to 4 days.

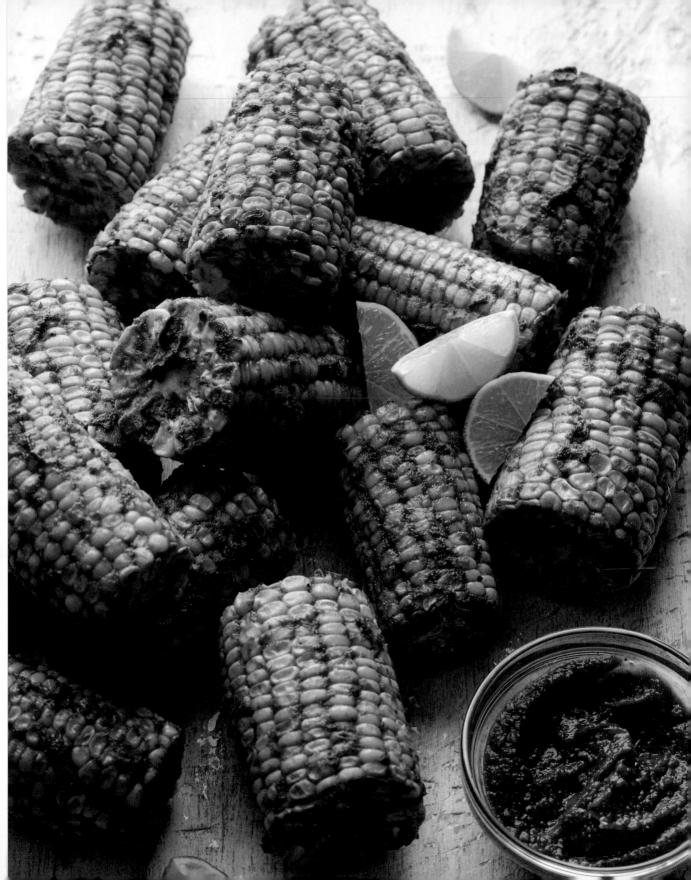

Masala-Baked Corn on the Cob

During corn season in India, pop-up street vendors fire up their coal grills to roast corn on the cob, which they flavor with cayenne pepper, lemon, and salt. In this recipe, I slather the corn with a masala curry paste, which turns the corn into an unusual and really flavorful treat. I bake the corn, but the corn is also delicious cooked on an outdoor grill.

Makes 8 corn cobs

Ready in 30 minutes

NOTE: For a Tex-Mex version of this corn, slather the corn with Chipotle Barbecue Sauce (page 333) instead of the Masala Curry Paste in this recipe.

8 corn cobs, shucked	Masala Curry Paste (recipe follows)	Limes, quartered, for serving

1. Preheat the oven to 450°F and place a baking rack on a baking sheet; or preheat a grill over high heat.
2. Smear 1 tablespoon of the paste on each corn cob and place the cobs on the baking rack or grill.
3. Bake the corn in the oven or cook it on the grill for 20 minutes. Remove the corn from the oven or grill. Serve with the lime wedges for squeezing onto each corn cob.

Masala Curry Paste

Masala paste, a combination of herbs and spices ground to a paste, is the basis of many Indian curries. The ingredients are traditionally ground using a mortar and pestle or a grinding stone, but I use a blender for convenience. Add this paste to sautéed vegetables, along with enough plant milk to make a creamy curry sauce.

Makes about ½ cup

Ready in 10 minutes

Nothing says "welcome" like a pot of vegetables or beans simmering on the stovetop with offerings for every season and from every corner of the world, soups and stews begging to be doubled. Take some to the office or enjoy this ultimate comfort food with your loved ones at home after a busy day.

6 | Soups and Stews

Sweet Potato Tortilla Soup

Makes about
6 cups

Ready in
35 minutes

Tortilla soup is one of my all-time favorite comfort foods. I make various styles of tortilla soup; this one brings together the rich flavor and creamy texture of sweet potatoes and the sweet, smoky flavors of roasted bell peppers and chipotle chiles. The soup is garnished with crispy tortilla strips. If you are using fresh corn, as opposed to frozen, try charring the corn in a dry sauté pan before adding it to the soup; the corn becomes chewy and adds another layer of flavor.

6 corn tortillas, cut into ¼-inch strips

1 medium sweet potato (about 12 ounces), cut into ½-inch dice

9 ounces jarred roasted red bell peppers, cored, seeded, and cut into ½-inch dice

2 Roma tomatoes or 1 large tomato (about 8 ounces), roughly chopped

4 ounces button mushrooms, trimmed and cut into ¾-inch dice (about 1 cup)

1 small yellow onion, cut into ¾-inch dice (about 1 cup)

4 medium garlic cloves, minced (about 2 teaspoons)

1 teaspoon ground cumin

1 teaspoon dried oregano (preferably Mexican oregano)

1 dried chipotle chile (about 2 ounces)

1 cup fresh or frozen corn kernels (from about 1 large cob)

½ tablespoon fresh lemon juice

Sea salt

2 scallions, thinly sliced (white and green parts, about ½ cup)

¼ cup finely chopped fresh cilantro

1. Preheat the oven to 350°F. Line a baking sheet with parchment paper.

2. Spread the tortilla strips on the baking sheet and bake until crispy and golden brown, 20 to 25 minutes, shaking the pan from time to time so the tortillas brown evenly. Set aside.

3. Meanwhile, place the sweet potato, bell peppers, tomatoes, mushrooms, onion, garlic, cumin, oregano, chile, and 4 cups water in a large soup pot or Dutch oven and bring to a boil over high heat. Reduce the heat to medium and simmer, covered, stirring occasionally, until the vegetables are tender, 20 to 25 minutes. Turn off the heat.

4. Remove and discard the chile and let the soup cool slightly. (If you put hot food in a blender, the heat will expand when you run the machine and the soup will explode out of the blender.)

5. Transfer the soup to a blender or food processor and blend until smooth. Pour the soup back into the pot. Add the corn, lemon juice, and salt to taste. Bring the soup to a boil over medium-high heat, stirring occasionally. Reduce the heat to medium and simmer for 5 minutes, to meld the flavors.

6. To serve, ladle the soup into individual bowls and garnish with the scallions, cilantro, and tortilla strips.

STORAGE: Let the soup cool to room temperature and transfer it to a container with a tight-fitting lid. Cover and refrigerate for up to 5 days or freeze for up to 6 weeks. Prepare the garnishes just before serving.

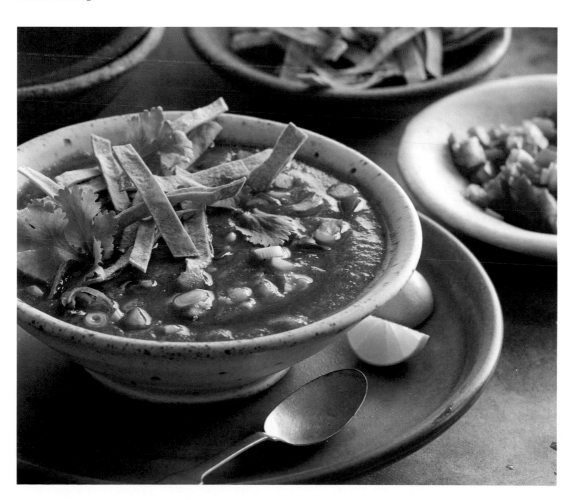

Lentil-Vegetable Tagine

Makes about
8 cups

Ready in
50 minutes

"I use a
vegetable
peeler to make
easy work
of peeling
tomatoes."

Tagine is a North African specialty named after the clay pot—a tagine—in which it is cooked. The pot has a conical lid that traps the moisture from the vegetables and condenses it back into the pot. Traditional tagine is made up of layers of vegetables cooked with herbs, spices, dried fruits, and preserved lemon (lemon preserved in salt). Here I use chopped fresh lemon rind, which imparts the same intense citrus flavor, in place of the preserved lemon. To simplify this recipe, use a smaller selection of vegetables.

NOTE: You will need an 8- to 10-inch sauté pan to make this. (I specify the size of the pan because if you use a larger pan, you won't have any of the delicious liquid left in the pan after cooking to spoon over the vegetables.)

½ medium yellow onion, cut into ¼-inch dice (about 1 cup)

4 medium garlic cloves, minced (about 2 teaspoons)

2 teaspoons grated peeled fresh ginger

1 medium tomato, peeled with a vegetable peeler and cut into ¼-inch dice (about ¾ cup)

2 tablespoons Ras el Hanout (recipe follows; or store-bought)

2 tablespoons roughly chopped fresh cilantro

1 cup red lentils, rinsed and drained

1 tablespoon finely chopped lemon rind

¼ teaspoon sea salt

¼ teaspoon ground black pepper

2 medium chayote squash (about 24 ounces), cut into 1-inch-thick, 1-inch-long wedges

1 red bell pepper, cored, seeded, and cut into ½-inch-thick, 2-inch-long strips (about 1 cup)

2 cups (1-inch) cauliflower florets (about 8 ounces)

Cooked rice, quinoa, or another grain; or Za'atar Spiced Pita Bread (page 299)

1. Combine the onion, garlic, ginger, and ¼ cup water in a 10-inch sauté pan and sauté over medium heat for about 10 minutes, until the onion is tender. Add the tomato, ras el hanout, and half of the cilantro and cook for 2 minutes to meld the

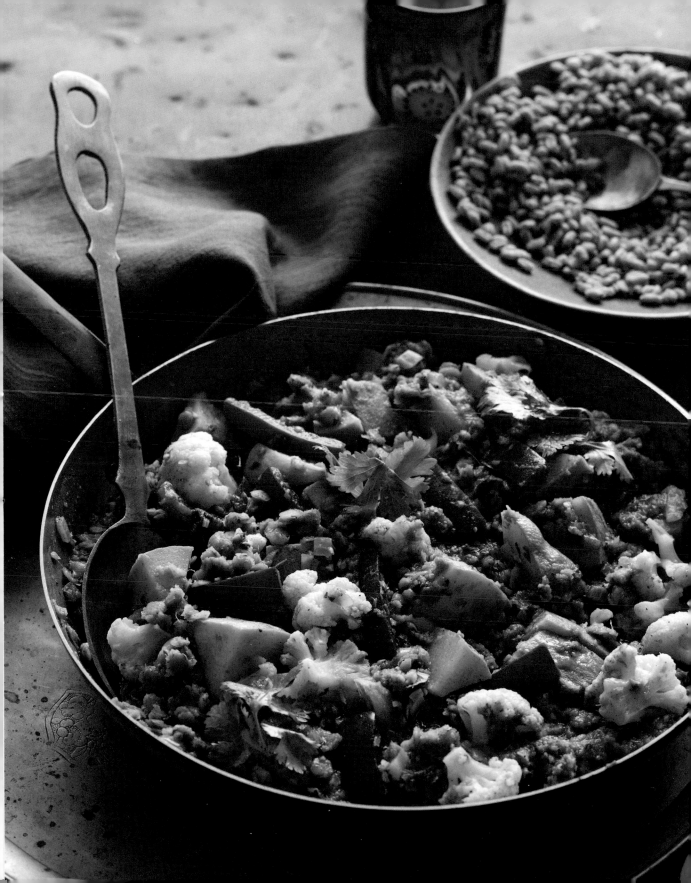

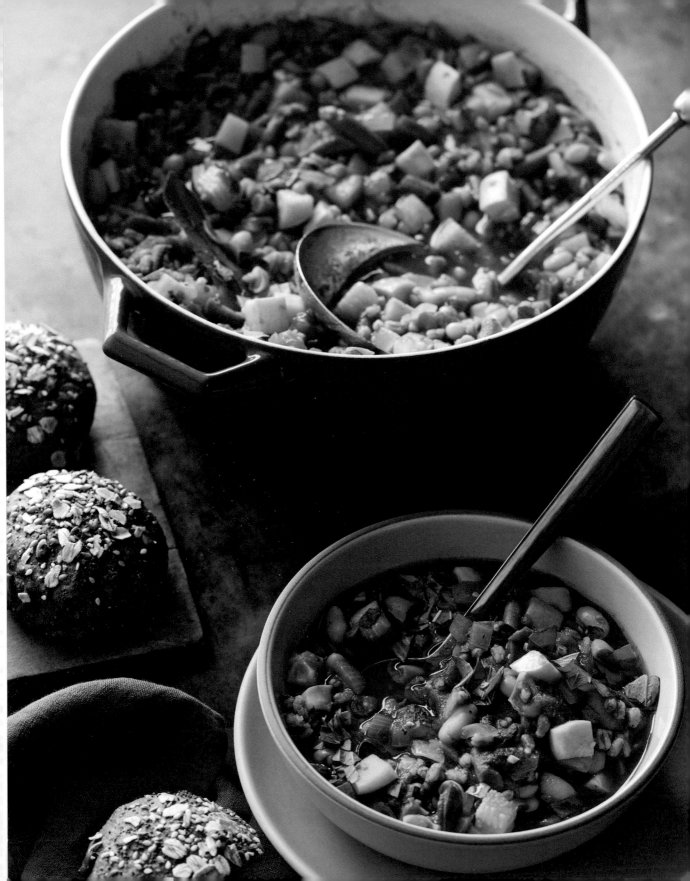

Farro Minestrone

This Italian vegetable soup comes to life with white beans, farro, and basil. Farro is an Italian variety of hulled wheat with an earthy flavor and chewy texture that feels just right for a minestrone. Other varieties of hulled wheat—such as spelt, emmer, and einkorn—are similar to farro and can be used instead.

Makes about
8 cups

Ready in
40 minutes

NOTE: Whole-grain farro takes a long time to cook, so if you can plan ahead, soak the grains overnight to reduce the cooking time by half.

½ cup whole-grain farro, rinsed and drained

1 medium yellow onion, cut into ½-inch dice (about 2 cups)

4 medium garlic cloves, minced (about 2 teaspoons)

1 dried bay leaf

3 cups 30-Minute Vegetable Stock (page 32; or oil free, low-sodium store-bought stock or water)

2 medium tomatoes, cut into ½-inch dice (about 2 cups)

2 medium zucchini (or yellow crookneck squash), cut into ½-inch dice (about 4 cups)

1 cup green beans (about 6 ounces), cut into ½-inch pieces

3 tablespoons tomato paste

1 teaspoon dried oregano

½ teaspoon dried thyme

1 (15-ounce) can white beans, rinsed and drained (about 1½ cups)

1 tablespoon white wine vinegar

Sea salt

Freshly ground black pepper

2 tablespoons finely chopped fresh basil

1. Combine the farro, onion, garlic, and bay leaf in a large pot or Dutch oven and cook over medium-low heat, stirring occasionally, for about 10 minutes, until the onion begins to brown, adding 1 to 2 more tablespoons of water as needed to keep the vegetables from sticking to the pan.

2. Add the stock, increase the heat to high, and bring to a boil. Reduce the heat to medium-low and simmer, covered, for about 20 minutes, until the farro is tender but still chewy. Add the tomatoes, zucchini, green beans, tomato paste, oregano, thyme, white beans, and vinegar, increase the heat to high, and return the soup to a boil. Reduce the heat to medium and simmer for about 5 minutes, until the vegetables are tender but still have a bite. Add salt and pepper to taste.

3. Serve warm, garnished with the basil.

STORAGE: Let the soup cool to room temperature and transfer it to a container with a tight-fitting lid. Cover and refrigerate for up to 5 days.

Korean Cold Noodle Soup

Makes about
6 cups plus about
4 cups noodles

Ready in
35 minutes

It's always exciting to discover a traditional dish that is made entirely from plants, such as kong guk su. I discovered this cold soy milk–based soup while researching Korean cuisine. I found it to be a simple yet exotic concept and decided to try a recipe I found online. The soup had wonderful, refreshing subtle flavors—a real delight! In my version, I use bright fresh vegetables, which add a color and a crunchy element to the original recipe.

6 ounces Thai-style brown rice noodles (or any whole-grain noodles, such as soba noodles, or whole-grain pasta)

6 cups chilled soy milk (or Quick Almond Milk, page 29; or store-bought plant milk)

3 medium garlic cloves, minced (about 1½ teaspoons)

1½ teaspoons grated peeled fresh ginger

Sea salt

Freshly ground black pepper

1 Persian cucumber, cut into fine matchsticks (about 1 cup)

½ medium red bell pepper, cored, seeded, and very thinly sliced (about ¾ cup)

½ medium carrot, peeled and cut into fine

matchsticks (about ½ cup)

½ cup cherry tomatoes, halved (about 1½ ounces)

2 teaspoons finely chopped fresh chives

1 tablespoon toasted sesame seeds (preferably black)

2 tablespoons pine nuts, lightly toasted (or roasted peanuts; optional)

1. Cook the noodles according to the package instructions. Drain in a colander and run cold water over the noodles to stop them from cooking. Set aside.

2. Combine the soy milk, garlic, and ginger in a deep bowl or a large pot. Add the noodles and refrigerate for at least 30 minutes and up to several hours to chill. Remove from the refrigerator and add salt and pepper to taste.

3. To serve, place the noodles in individual bowls. Ladle the soup over the noodles. Top with the cucumber, bell pepper, carrot, and tomatoes and garnish with the chives, sesame seeds, and pine nuts (if you're using them).

STORAGE: Store the soy milk mixture, noodles, and vegetables in separate containers. Cover and refrigerate for up to 3 days.

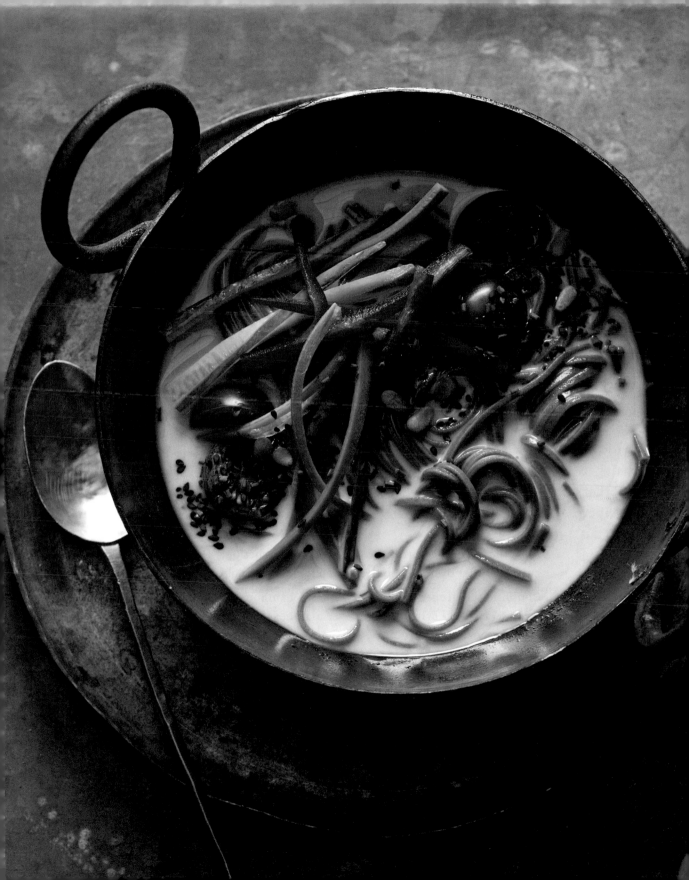

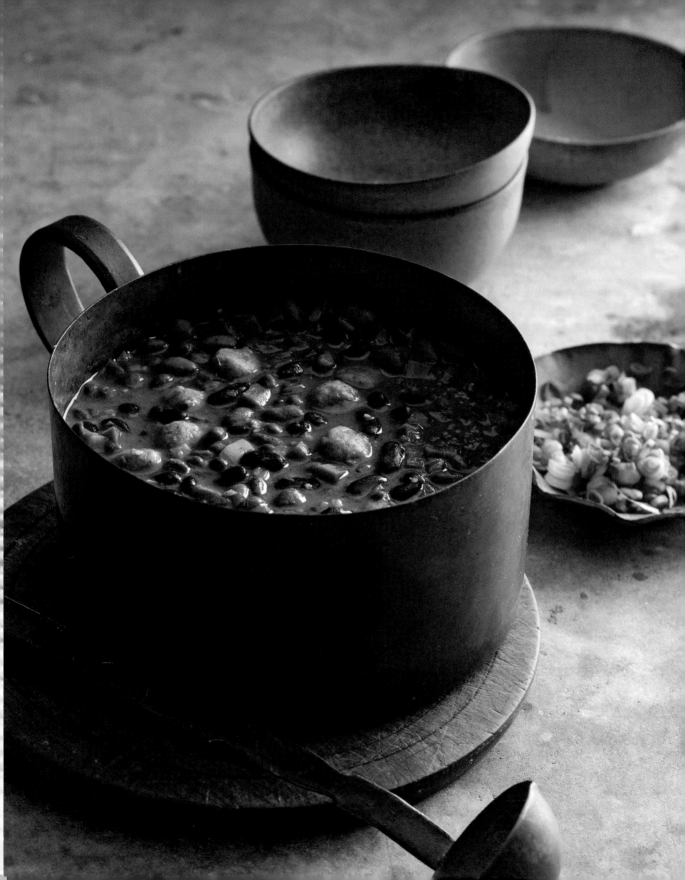

Stewpea: Jamaican Mixed Vegetable and Dumpling Stew

When we arrived at our friend Donovan Green's home for dinner one night a couple of years ago, we were thrilled to learn that his mom, Velma, had cooked us a Jamaican meal. We were treated to a vegan version of stewpea, a delicious combination of beans, herbs, spices, and tender dumplings. The meal was so good, we almost couldn't stop eating. Thankfully, Velma had a lot of experience serving her stew and was ready with a huge pot. In this version of stewpea, I stay true to the herbs and spices and use pinto and kidney beans. The bite-size dumplings in this rich stew are a nice treat. Scotch bonnet peppers are small yellowish orange chiles native to the Caribbean. If you can't find them, use habanero peppers, which look almost identical, instead. For gluten-free dumplings, use a combination of oat flour and amaranth flour in place of the whole-wheat flour.

Makes about
6 cups

Ready in
50 minutes

½ medium yellow onion, cut into ¼-inch dice (about 1 cup)

4 medium garlic cloves, minced (about 2 teaspoons)

½ tablespoon grated peeled fresh ginger

2 (15-ounce) cans pinto beans, rinsed and drained (about 3 cups)

1 (15-ounce) can kidney beans, rinsed and drained (about 1½ cups)

2 medium carrots, peeled and cut into ¼-inch dice (about 1 cup)

1 medium tomato, cut into ½-inch dice (about 6 ounces)

1 tablespoon finely chopped fresh thyme (or 2 teaspoons dried thyme)

¾ teaspoon ground allspice

Half of a small Scotch bonnet pepper (or habanero), seeded and finely chopped

¼ cup whole-wheat flour (or 2 tablespoons oat flour and 2 tablespoons amaranth flour)

½ cup unsweetened, unflavored plant milk

1 tablespoon fresh lime juice

Sea salt

2 scallions, thinly sliced (white and green parts; about ½ cup)

1. Combine the onion, garlic, ginger, and ¼ cup water in a large saute pan and cook over medium heat, stirring frequently, until the onion is tender and starts to

brown, about 10 minutes, adding 1 to 2 more tablespoons of water as needed to keep the vegetables from sticking to the pan. Add the pinto beans, kidney beans, carrots, tomato, thyme, allspice, pepper, and 4 cups water and bring the water to a boil over high heat. Reduce the heat to medium and simmer for 10 minutes to begin to soften the vegetables.

2. Meanwhile, in a medium bowl, combine the flour and 2 tablespoons water and stir to form a dough. Drop the dough into the stew in ¼-teaspoon portions. Add the milk and cook for about 20 minutes, until the vegetables are tender and the soup is thick. Turn off the heat. Stir in the lime juice and salt to taste.

3. Serve warm, garnished with the scallions.

STORAGE: Let the stew cool to room temperature. Transfer to a container with a tight-fitting lid. Cover and refrigerate for up to 3 days or freeze for up to 1 month.

Ethiopian Red Lentil Stew

Rahel Ethiopian Vegan Cuisine in Los Angeles serves some of the best Ethiopian food I've ever tasted. The owner, Rahel Woldmedhin, is happy to serve oil-free dishes upon request. After Rahel shared some of her tips for Ethiopian cooking with me, I was inspired to create this berbere-spiced red lentil stew. Berbere is an East African spice blend that usually includes allspice, cinnamon, cloves, cardamom, coriander, fenugreek, nutmeg, and turmeric. I provide a recipe for the blend, but you can also find it in supermarkets, health food stores, or online.

Makes about
8 cups

Ready in
45 minutes

1 medium red onion, cut into ¼-inch dice (about 2 cups)

12 medium garlic cloves, minced (about 2 tablespoons)

2 tablespoons grated peeled fresh ginger

2 to 3 tablespoons Berbere

Spice Blend (recipe follows; or store-bought)

½ teaspoon ground cardamom

2 cups red lentils, rinsed and drained

2 cups (½-inch diced) green cabbage (about 5 ounces)

1 tablespoon fresh lemon juice

Sea salt

1 tablespoon finely chopped fresh cilantro (or parsley)

Cooked grains (such as brown rice or quinoa)

1. Combine the onion, garlic, ginger, and 1 cup water in a large sauté pan and cook, covered, over medium heat for about 10 minutes, until the onion is tender. Add the spice blend and cardamom and cook for 2 minutes to toast the spices.

2. Add the lentils and 4 cups water and bring the water to a boil over high heat. Reduce the heat to medium and simmer until the lentils are completely cooked, about 20 minutes, stirring occasionally.

3. Add the cabbage, lemon juice, and salt to taste and cook for 10 to 15 minutes, until the cabbage wilts. Stir in the cilantro.

4. Serve warm, spooned over the cooked grains and garnished with the cilantro.

STORAGE: Let the stew cool to room temperature. Transfer to a container with a tight-fitting lid. Cover and refrigerate for up to 3 days or freeze for up to 1 month.

Caldo Verde: Portuguese Potato and Kale Soup

Makes about
8 cups

Ready in
35 minutes

I often ask my friends to recommend vegetarian (or easily adaptable to vegetarian) dishes. A Portuguese friend suggested caldo verde, a simple soup packed with potatoes and greens. This recipe, which utilizes kale, reminds me of how scrumptious a dish with only a few of the right ingredients can be.

1 small yellow onion, cut into ¼-inch dice (about 1 cup)

4 medium garlic cloves, minced (about 2 teaspoons)

1 dried bay leaf

1 (3-inch) cinnamon stick

6 cups 30-Minute Vegetable Stock (page 32; or oil-free, low-sodium store-bought stock or water)

2 pounds potatoes (any variety), cut into ¾-inch dice (about 8 cups)

1 carrot, peeled and sliced ¼ inch thick (about ½ cup)

1 bunch kale, stems removed and discarded, leaves shredded (about 4 cups)

Sea salt

⅛ teaspoon ground black pepper

1. Combine the onion, garlic, bay leaf, and cinnamon stick in a large pot or Dutch oven. Add ¼ cup water and sauté over medium-low heat for about 10 minutes, stirring occasionally, until the onion is tender, adding 1 to 2 more tablespoons of water as needed to keep the vegetables from sticking to the pan.

2. Add the stock, potatoes, and carrot and bring to a boil over high heat. Reduce the heat to medium and simmer for 10 to 15 minutes, until the potatoes are tender when pierced with a fork. Remove the cinnamon stick and bay leaf. Using a potato masher or a hand blender, coarsely mash the vegetables, leaving the soup chunky.

3. Add the kale and 1 to 2 cups water, or enough to make a soupy consistency, and cook for 5 to 10 minutes, until the kale is cooked to your liking. Turn off the heat and stir in the salt to taste and pepper. Serve warm.

STORAGE: Let the soup cool to room temperature. Transfer to a container with a tight-fitting lid. Cover and refrigerate for up to 3 days or freeze for up to 1 month.

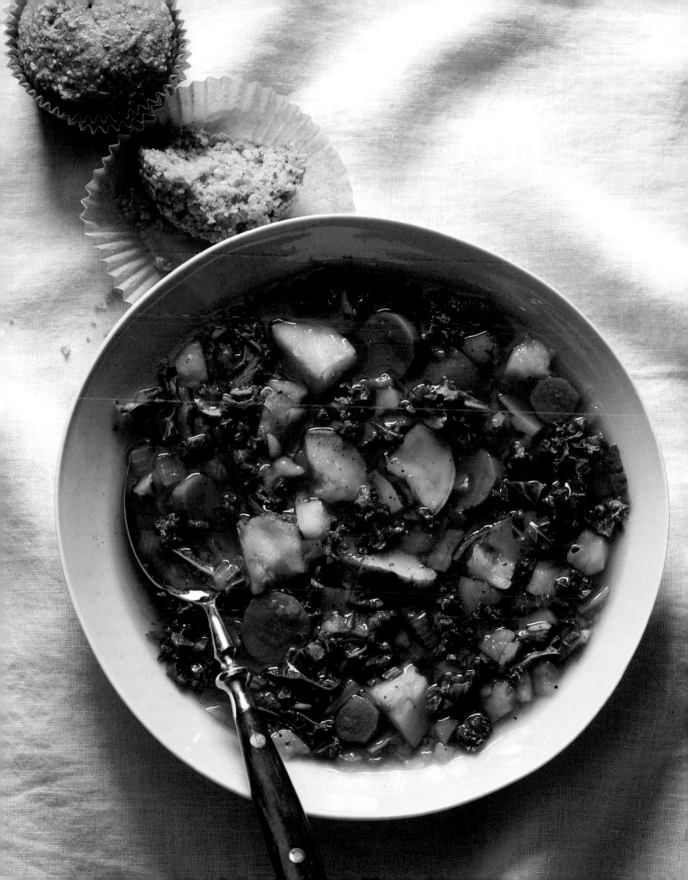

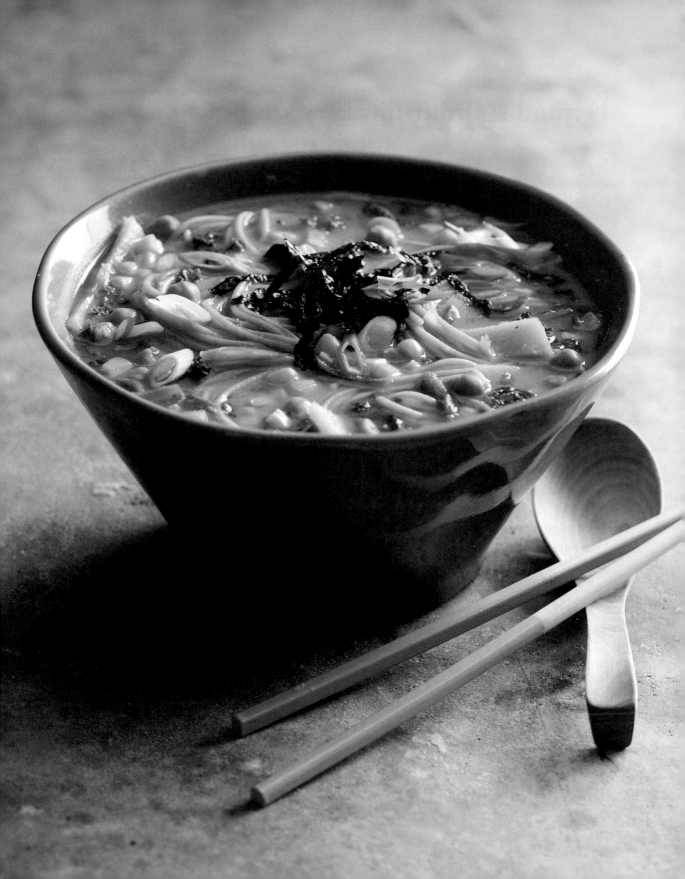

Spicy Miso Ramen

There are countless regional versions of Japanese ramen, including some like this one that are thick and creamy. It is sprinkled with togarashi, a Japanese spice blend, which you can find at Asian grocery stores, many conventional supermarkets, and online.

Makes about
8 cups plus about
4 cups noodles

Ready in
30 minutes

6 ounces long whole-grain noodles (such as spaghetti, Thai-style brown rice noodles, or soba or udon noodles)

2 tablespoons chickpea flour

¼ cup miso (any type)

8 ounces thinly sliced bamboo shoots (about 2 cups)

½ tablespoon grated peeled fresh ginger

3 medium garlic cloves, minced (about ½ tablespoon)

Dash of togarashi (or 1 teaspoon hot sauce, such as sriracha or sambal olek)

½ bunch kale, stems removed and discarded, coarsely chopped (about 2 cups)

1 (15-ounce) can chickpeas, rinsed and drained (about 1½ cups)

1 cup fresh or frozen corn kernels (from about 1 large cob)

1 medium carrot, peeled and grated on the large holes of a box grater (about ½ cup)

2 scallions, thinly sliced on the bias (white and green parts; about ½ cup)

1 sheet nori, cut into thin ribbons

1. Cook the noodles according to the package instructions. Drain in a colander and run cold water over the noodles to stop them from cooking. Set aside.

2. Combine the flour, miso, and ½ cup water in a small bowl and stir with a fork until no lumps remain. (This mixture is called a slurry.) Set aside.

3. Combine the bamboo shoots, ginger, garlic, and 6 cups water in a large sauté pan and bring to a boil over high heat. Reduce the heat to medium-low and simmer for 5 minutes. Stir in the slurry and togarashi and simmer, stirring occasionally, for 5 to 7 minutes, until the soup thickens slightly. Add the kale, chickpeas, corn, and carrot and cook for 2 to 3 minutes, until the kale wilts slightly. Turn off the heat.

4. To serve, place the noodles in large individual bowls. Ladle the broth and the vegetables over the noodles and garnish with scallions and nori.

STORAGE: Let the soup cool to room temperature. Store the soup and noodles in separate containers. Cover and refrigerate for up to 3 days.

Casseroles, lasagnas, and hearty savory pies may take some time, but the good news is, the oven does all the work—and creates all the magic. So sit back in anticipation, and enjoy the wonderful scents coming from the kitchen.

7 | Baked Entrees

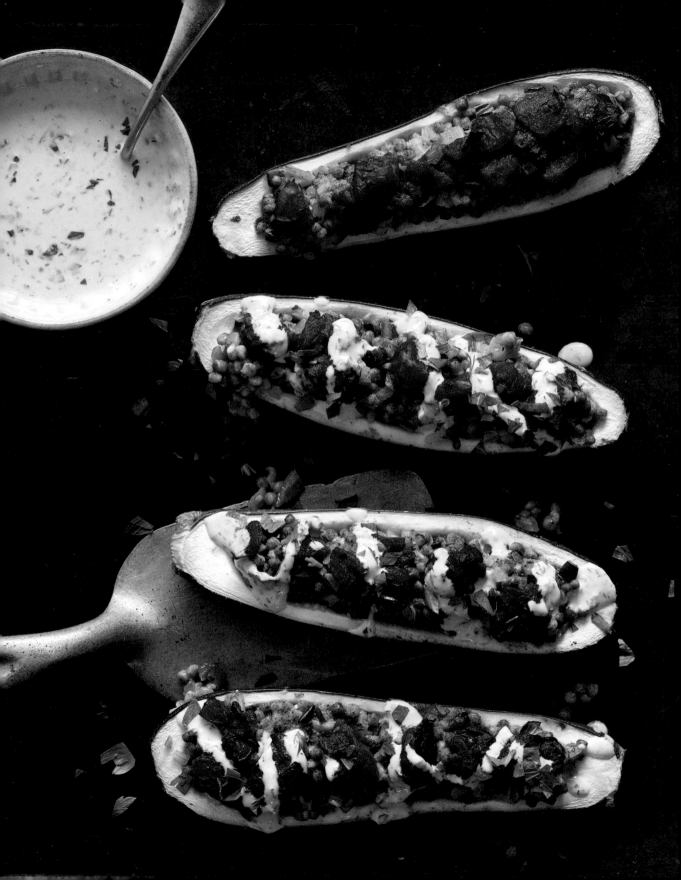

Stuffed Zucchini Boats with Israeli Couscous and Parsley Tahini Sauce

Israeli couscous, also called pearl couscous, is a small pearl-shaped pasta. In this recipe, I sauté the cooked pasta with a mix of flavorful vegetables, and use it to stuff zucchini "boats." I use Mexican poblano pepper in this Middle Eastern casserole because it adds a distinct, pungent flavor to the dish. Sumac is a seasoning common in Middle Eastern cooking; you will find it at specialty food stores and Middle Eastern markets. The dish will taste good without sumac, so no worries if you can't find it.

Makes 8 zucchini boats

Ready in 50 minutes

NOTE: You can use this stuffing to fill any squash, including large pattypan squashes in the summer and delicata or acorn squash in the winter.

4 large zucchini (or yellow squash; about 2 pounds)

¾ cup whole-wheat Israeli couscous

½ medium yellow onion, cut into ¼-inch dice (about 1 cup)

1 medium poblano chile (or red or green bell pepper), cored, seeded, and cut into ¼-inch dice (about 1 cup)

9 medium garlic cloves, minced (about 1½ tablespoons)

1 teaspoon ground cumin

1 teaspoon ground sumac (optional)

¼ teaspoon cayenne pepper

2 tablespoons finely chopped fresh parsley

½ tablespoon finely grated lemon zest

1 tablespoon fresh lemon juice

Sea salt

1 (15-ounce) can sodium-free or low-sodium diced tomatoes (preferably fire-roasted; about 1½ cups)

¼ cup Parsley Tahini Sauce (page 341)

1. Preheat the oven to 400°F.

2. Cut the zucchini in half lengthwise. Using a small spoon, scoop the seeds and flesh out of the zucchini to create zucchini "boats." Chop up the scraps and put them into a large saucepan.

3. Place the zucchini boats in a baking dish. Cover the dish with foil and bake for 20 minutes.

3. Meanwhile, to make the filling, place a steamer basket in a medium saucepan and add 1 to 2 inches of water to the pan. Bring the water to a simmer over medium-high heat. Place the sweet potatoes in the steamer, cover, and steam until tender when pierced with a fork, about 10 minutes. Uncover. Transfer the sweet potatoes to a bowl and smash coarsely with a fork or potato masher.

4. While the sweet potatoes are steaming, in a large sauté pan, combine the onion, bell peppers, garlic, and ¼ cup water and cook over medium heat, stirring frequently, until the onion is tender, about 10 minutes, adding 1 to 2 more tablespoons of water as needed to keep the vegetables from sticking to the pan. Add the beans, corn, lime juice, and salt to taste and stir to combine.

5. Cut the edges off of the tortillas to form 1 large square from each tortilla. (Reserve the scraps; toast them in a 350°F oven for about 20 minutes, until they're golden brown and crispy, and toss them into soups and salads or munch on them.)

6. Spread 1½ cups of the enchilada sauce over the bottom of a large (9-by-13-inch) baking dish. Place 6 tortilla squares in the baking dish, leaving as much space between the squares as you can. Spread the mashed sweet potatoes over the tortillas, dividing them evenly. Drizzle or dollop half of the potato "cheese" sauce over the sweet potatoes. Spread the vegetable mixture in an even layer over the sauce. Place a tortilla square on each stack to cover it. Drizzle the remaining enchilada sauce over the tortillas and spoon the remaining potato "cheese" sauce over the enchilada sauce. (The enchiladas can be assembled to this point in advance. Cover the dish tightly with plastic wrap. Refrigerate for up to 1 day and freeze for up to 1 month. Bake the refrigerated enchilada stacks in a 400°F oven according to the recipe; bake frozen enchilada stacks for 10 to 20 minutes longer.)

7. Place the enchilada stacks in the oven for 20 minutes to heat them through. Remove from the oven and set aside to allow them to cool for 5 to 10 minutes before serving. Serve hot, garnished with the scallion.

STORAGE: Cool the stacks to room temperature, then cover tightly with plastic wrap and refrigerate for up to 3 days. Uncover and warm in a preheated 350°F oven until heated through.

Potato Panade with Garlic and Fresh Thyme

I love the combination of potatoes, bread, and a creamy sauce, which is common in French cooking; this baked entree combines all three into a warm, richly flavored casserole. If you're a greens lover, you may want to double (or even triple) the amount of spinach in the recipe.

Makes 1 9-by-13-inch baking dish

Ready in 1 hour

NOTE: You will need a 9-by-13-inch baking dish to make this.

5 slices whole-grain bread, cut into quarters (about 4 cups)

2 medium russet potatoes (about 16 ounces), scrubbed and sliced into ¼-inch-thick disks

4 medium carrots, sliced ¼ inch thick (about 2 cups)

1 medium yellow onion, thinly sliced (about 2 cups)

6 medium garlic cloves, minced (about 1 tablespoon)

5 cups unsweetened, unflavored plant milk

¼ cup unbleached all-purpose flour (or whole-wheat flour)

3 tablespoons nutritional yeast

2 teaspoons finely chopped fresh thyme

½ teaspoon freshly grated nutmeg

2 cups fresh spinach (or chard or kale), finely chopped (about 2 ounces)

1 tablespoon fresh lemon juice

Sea salt

Freshly ground black pepper

1. Preheat the oven to 400°F.

2. Spread the bread pieces on a baking sheet and bake in the oven for about 10 minutes, until crispy, turning them halfway through the cooking time with tongs so they crisp evenly. Remove from the oven.

3. Place a steamer basket in a medium saucepan and add 1 to 2 inches of water to the pan. Cover and bring the water to a simmer over medium-high heat. Place the potatoes in the steamer, cover, and steam until tender when pierced with a fork, 15 to 20 minutes. Uncover. Transfer the potatoes to a large bowl and set aside until they are cool enough to handle.

4. Put the carrots, onion, and garlic in a large pot or Dutch oven and cook over me-

dium heat for about 10 minutes, stirring occasionally and adding 1 to 2 more tablespoons of water as needed to keep the vegetables from sticking to the pan, until the vegetables are tender.

5. Meanwhile, combine the milk, flour, yeast, thyme, and nutmeg in a mixing bowl and whisk to combine. Pour the milk mixture into the pan with the vegetables and cook for about 10 minutes, stirring to keep the milk from sticking to the pan, until the sauce thickens to a soup consistency. Stir in the spinach and lemon juice. Turn off the heat and stir in salt and pepper to taste.

6. Lay half of the toasted bread on the bottom of a 9-by 13-inch baking dish. Lay half of the sliced potatoes over the bread and pour half of the vegetable sauce over the bread and potatoes. Repeat, making another layer with the remaining bread and potatoes and cover with the remaining sauce.

7. Bake the panade in the oven for about 30 minutes, until the sauce bubbles and the top is golden brown. Remove from the oven and set aside to cool for at least 5 minutes before cutting.

STORAGE: Cool the panade to room temperature, then cover tightly with plastic wrap or place in individual portions in covered containers. Refrigerate for up to 3 days or freeze for up to 1 month. Heat in a preheated 350°F oven until warmed through.

Australian Pot Pie

The rising popularity of savory pies in the United States is a welcome trend. In large part, we have the Aussies to thank for this recent emergence, with savory pie shops owned by Aussies opening in many cities. Pies provide awesome texture, with a nice crunch on the outside and a delicious soft filling on the inside. It's enough to make a person smile from here to Sydney. In this pie, I use lots of beans and vegetables, seasoned with fresh herbs, in the filling. The secret of the flaky crust, if you will believe it, is mashed potatoes.

Makes 1 9- or
9½-inch pie

Ready in 1 hour,
40 minutes

NOTE: This pot pie may be made gluten-free by substituting the whole-wheat flour with oat and sorghum flour.

NOTE: You will need a 9- or 9½-inch pie plate to make this.

For the Crust

1½ pounds russet potatoes, peeled and cut into large pieces (about 4 cups)

1 cup whole-wheat flour (or ¾ cup oat flour and ¼ cup sorghum flour)

3 tablespoons almond flour

2 tablespoons flaxseed meal (preferably golden)

For the Filling

5 ounces white button mushrooms, trimmed and sliced (about 2 cups)

1 medium yellow onion, cut into ½-inch dice (about 1 cup)

1 celery stalk, cut into ½-inch dice (about ½ cup)

8 medium garlic cloves, minced (about 1 tablespoon plus 1 teaspoon)

¼ cup whole-wheat flour (or oat flour)

2 tablespoons tomato paste

2 tablespoons red wine vinegar

4 cups frozen mixed small vegetables (such as carrots, peas, and green beans; or another blend; about 24 ounces)

1 (15-ounce) can cannellini beans, rinsed and drained (about 1½ cups)

1 tablespoon finely chopped fresh thyme (or ½ tablespoon dried)

1 tablespoon finely chopped fresh rosemary (or ½ tablespoon dried)

Sea salt

Freshly ground black pepper

1. Preheat the oven to 400°F.

2. Place a steamer basket in a medium saucepan and add 1 to 2 inches of water to

the pan. Bring the water to a simmer over medium-high heat. Place the potatoes in the steamer, cover, and steam for 15 to 20 minutes, until they are tender when pierced with a fork. Remove the potatoes from the steamer and set aside to cool slightly.

3. In a food processor fitted with the dough blade or the bowl of a stand mixer fitted with the paddle attachment, mix the potatoes until they are coarsely mashed. Add the whole-wheat flour, almond flour, flaxseed meal, and ¼ cup water and mix to combine. The texture of the dough will be crumbly and dry, but it should come together when pressed with your hands. If the dough is too dry to do this, add just enough water to bring it together.

4. Using a rubber spatula, transfer the dough onto a piece of plastic wrap laid out on a flat surface. Pat the dough into a ball and divide it into 2 portions. Set one portion aside and cover the second portion with a second sheet of plastic wrap. Using a rolling pin, roll the dough out to an 11-inch round. Remove the top sheet of plastic wrap, reserving it, and flip the sheet of dough onto a 9½-inch pie dish. Peel off the plastic wrap, reserving it, and pat the dough to line the bottom and sides of the dish.

5. Place the pie shell in the oven to bake for 10 minutes. Remove the pie shell from the oven and set aside.

6. While the pie shell is baking, put the second portion of dough on one of the reserved sheets of plastic wrap. Cover with the second reserved sheet of plastic wrap and roll the dough into a 11-inch round. Carefully place it in the refrigerator.

7. Meanwhile, to make the filling, combine the mushrooms, onion, celery, garlic, and ½ cup of water in a medium saucepan and cook over medium heat until the vegetables are tender, about 10 minutes.

8. Mix the flour, tomato paste, vinegar, and 1 cup water in a small bowl. Add the mixture to the pan with the onion and mushrooms. Add the frozen mixed vegetables, beans, thyme, and rosemary and cook over medium heat, stirring occasionally, until the gravy thickens, about 7 minutes. Add salt and pepper to taste.

9. Pour the filling into the baked pie crust. Remove the round of dough from the refrigerator. Remove and discard the top sheet of plastic and flip the dough to lay it on top of the filling. Remove and discard the second sheet of plastic. Use your fingers or the tines of a fork to seal the top crust to the bottom crust. Using a small sharp knife, cut a slit in the top crust so the hot air can escape.

10. Place the pie on a baking sheet and bake in the oven until the crust is lightly browned, 30 to 40 minutes. Remove from the oven and let the pie rest for at least 5 minutes before serving. Cut the pie into 8 equal slices and serve hot.

STORAGE: Cool the pie to room temperature, then cover tightly with plastic wrap or place in individual portions in covered containers and refrigerate for up to 3 days or freeze for up to 1 month. Heat in a preheated 350°F oven until warmed through.

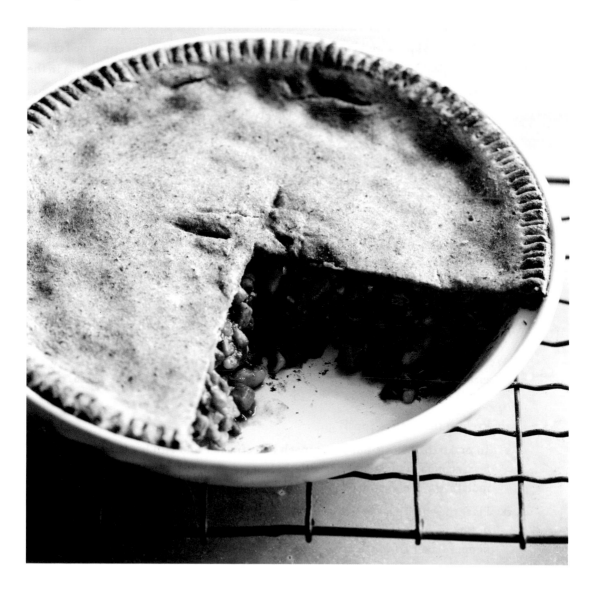

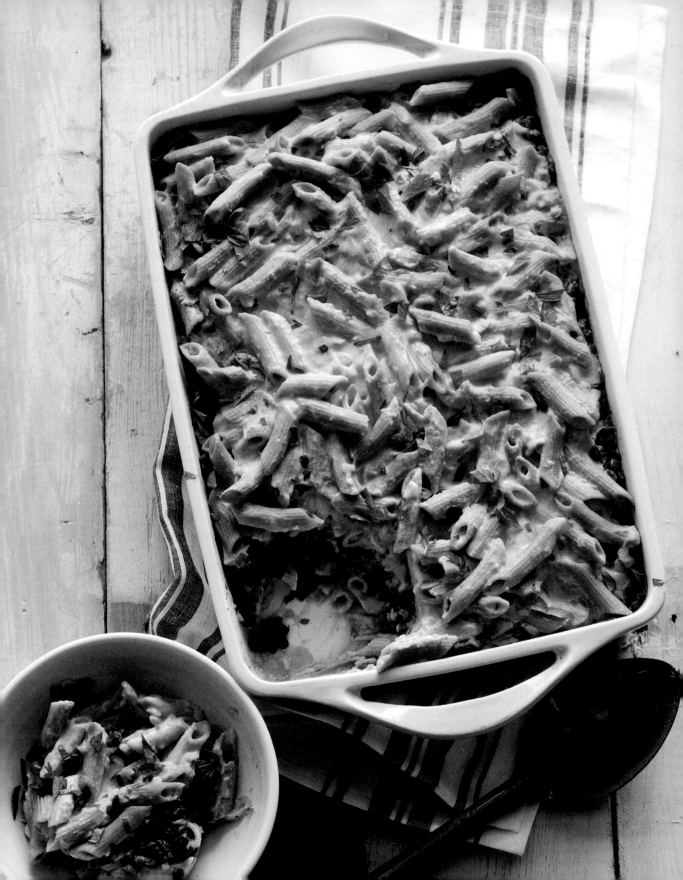

Pastitsio: Greek Pasta with Lentils and Potato "Cheese" Sauce

Since Brian is part Greek, I like to cook Greek recipes, such as pastitsio, a layered pasta dish similar to lasagna. In this recipe, whole-grain pasta is layered with spiced lentils and a creamy "cheese" sauce. It's one of my favorite baked dishes in this book.

Makes 1 9-by-13-inch baking dish

Ready in 50 minutes

NOTE: You will need a 9-by-13-inch (or similar size) baking dish to make this.

1 yellow onion, cut into ¼-inch dice (about 2 cups)

6 medium garlic cloves, minced (about 1 tablespoon)

1 (28-ounce) can sodium-free or low-sodium diced tomatoes (about 3 cups)

3 (15-ounce) cans lentils, rinsed and drained (about 4½ cups)

2 tablespoons fresh lemon juice

½ teaspoon ground cinnamon

½ teaspoon ground nutmeg

½ teaspoon ground black pepper

Sea salt

1 pound whole-grain penne or rigatoni (or another short-shape pasta)

2 cups unsweetened, unflavored plant milk

½ cup nutritional yeast

¼ cup brown rice flour

Doubled recipe of Potato "Cheese" Sauce (page 33; about 4 cups)

1. Preheat the oven to 375°F.

2. Combine the onion, garlic, and ¼ cup water in a large saucepan and cook over medium heat, stirring frequently, until the onion is tender, about 10 minutes, adding 1 to 2 more tablespoons of water as needed to keep the vegetables from sticking to the pan. Add the tomatoes, lentils, lemon juice, cinnamon, nutmeg, and pepper and cook until the liquid from the tomatoes has been cooked off, about 10 minutes. Add salt to taste.

3. Cook the pasta according to the package instructions, undercooking it by about 2 minutes, as it will cook further when baked. Transfer the cooked pasta to a large bowl.

medium heat, stirring occasionally, for 10 minutes. Add the kidney beans and cauliflower and cook for 5 minutes, or until the cauliflower begins to soften.

4. Combine the stock and flour in a small bowl and whisk until no lumps remain. (This mixture is called a slurry.) Pour the slurry into the pan with the vegetables and mix well. Cook for 3 to 4 minutes, until the sauce thickens. Add the lemon juice and salt to taste and stir to combine.

5. Transfer the vegetables to a 7-by-11-inch (or similar size) baking dish. Spread the mashed potatoes in an even layer over the vegetables.

6. Put the baking dish on a baking sheet to capture any drippings and bake in the oven for 30 to 40 minutes, until the top is golden brown. Remove from the oven and set the pie aside to cool slightly before scooping into it.

STORAGE: Cool the shepherd's pie to room temperature, then cover tightly with plastic wrap or place in individual portions in covered containers. Refrigerate for up to 3 days or freeze for up to 1 month. Heat in a preheated 350°F oven until warmed through.

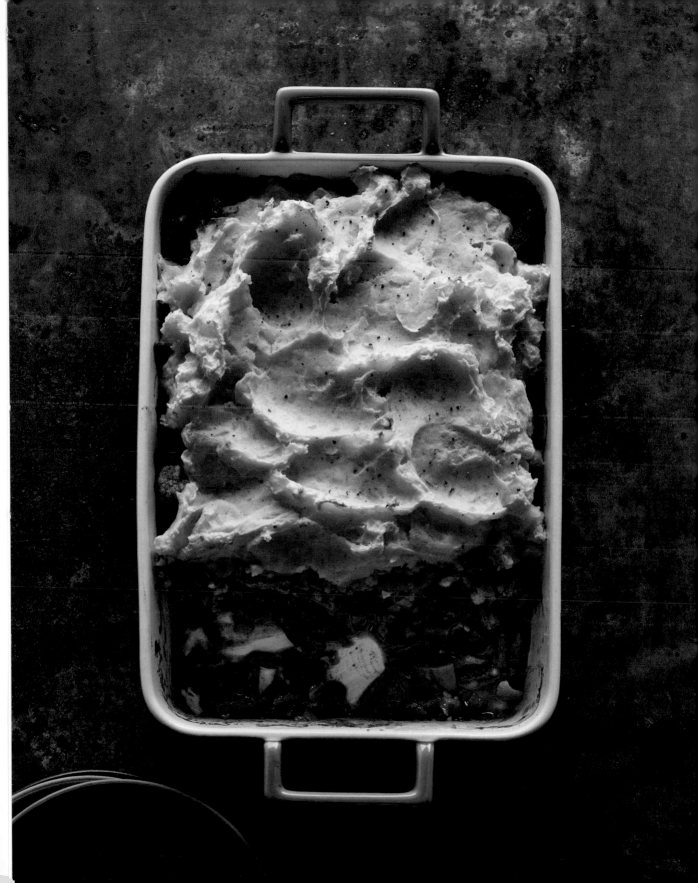

There's something about noodles. From Japanese soba and Chinese lo mein to Italian penne and good old-fashioned spaghetti, those strands and shapes are the definition of comfort food—wherever in the world they are found.

8 | Pasta and Noodles

Penne with Eggplant-Lentil "Bolognese" Sauce

Pasta with Bolognese, or meat, sauce is a popular Italian pasta dish. I enjoy creating plant-based versions of Bolognese sauce because I like the way the hearty sauce complements the pasta. In this recipe I use a combination of eggplant and lentils to make this very special sauce.

1 small yellow onion, cut into large pieces (about 1 cup)

2 celery stalks, cut into large pieces

1 medium carrot, peeled and cut into large pieces

6 medium garlic cloves (or about 1 tablespoon minced garlic)

8 ounces mushrooms, trimmed and cut into large pieces (about 3 cups)

1 small eggplant (about 1 pound), cut into large pieces

1 tablespoon dried rosemary

1 (15-ounce) can sodium-free or low-sodium lentils (about 1½ cups)

1 (28-ounce) can sodium-free or low-sodium tomato sauce (about 2½ cups)

Sea salt

Freshly ground black pepper

8 ounces whole-grain penne (or another shape of whole-grain pasta)

Frozen Cashew Chickpea "Cheese" (page 35) or nutritional yeast

1 tablespoon finely chopped fresh Italian parsley

1. Working in two batches, put the onion, celery, carrot, and garlic into the bowl of a food processor and pulse to mince the vegetables. Transfer the vegetables to a large sauté pan and repeat, mincing the second batch of vegetables in the same way and adding them to the pan with the first batch. Put the mushrooms into the food processor and pulse to mince them. Add them to the pan with the other vegetables. Put the eggplant into the food processor and pulse to mince. Add it to the pan. Add the rosemary and ¼ cup water and sauté for 10 to 15 minutes, stirring occasionally, to soften the vegetables.

2. Add the lentils and tomato sauce and cook for about 10 minutes to allow the flavors to merge. Add salt and pepper to taste.

3. Meanwhile, cook the pasta according to the package instructions. Drain in a colander and set aside.

4. To serve, place the pasta in a serving bowl and pour the sauce over it. Grate the "cheese" over the pasta or sprinkle it with nutritional yeast. Garnish with the parsley and serve.

STORAGE: Refrigerate the sauce in an airtight container for up to 5 days or freeze for up to 1 month. Serve with freshly cooked pasta.

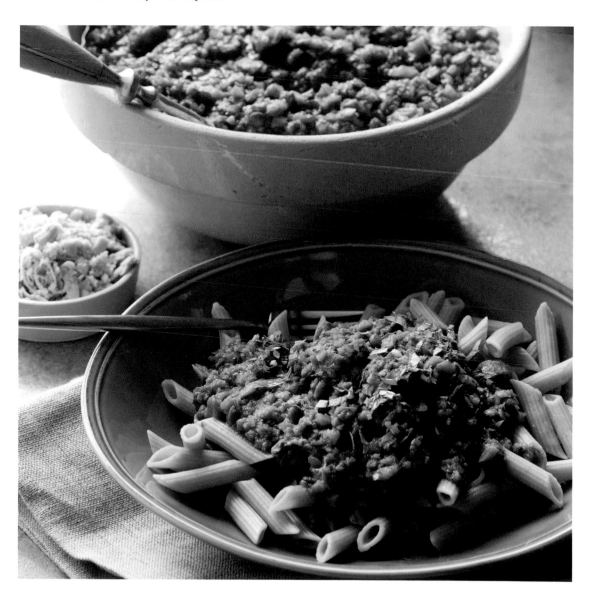

Spaghetti Tricolore with Myrna's Marinara Sauce

Makes about
6 cups

Ready in
25 minutes

Maybe it was Halloween that got into me, but I had the idea one day that veggies, deep down, want to dress up like pasta. So that day I made a bowl of spaghetti, added spiralized zucchini and carrots, and tossed them all with marinara sauce. Sure enough, it looked like a dish of orange, white, and green spaghetti. It's a really delicious and easy meal, especially if you already have marinara sauce on hand.

NOTE: You can buy spiralized zucchini and carrots in many grocery stores. If you want to make your own, you can buy an inexpensive handheld spiralizer. If you're really excited about spiralizing, you can invest in a more expensive countertop spiralizer.

6 ounces whole-grain spaghetti

2 cups Myrna's Marinara Sauce (page 34; or store-bought oil-free marinara sauce)

6 ounces spiralized zucchini (about 1 medium zucchini; about 2 cups)

6 ounces spiralized carrot (about 2 medium carrots; about 2 cups)

1 (15-ounce) can chickpeas, drained and rinsed (about 1 ½ cups)

¼ cup pitted, sliced black olives (optional)

¼ cup fresh basil leaves

1. Cook the spaghetti according to the package instructions. Drain in a colander and set aside.

2. Meanwhile, heat the sauce over medium heat in a large sauté pan until it's warmed through. Add the spiralized zucchini and carrot, chickpeas, and cooked pasta and stir to combine. Increase the heat to medium-high and cook for 5 to 7 minutes, until the carrot softens slightly. Stir in the olives (if you're using them).

3. Garnish with the basil and serve right away.

STORAGE: Refrigerate in an airtight container for up to 4 days.

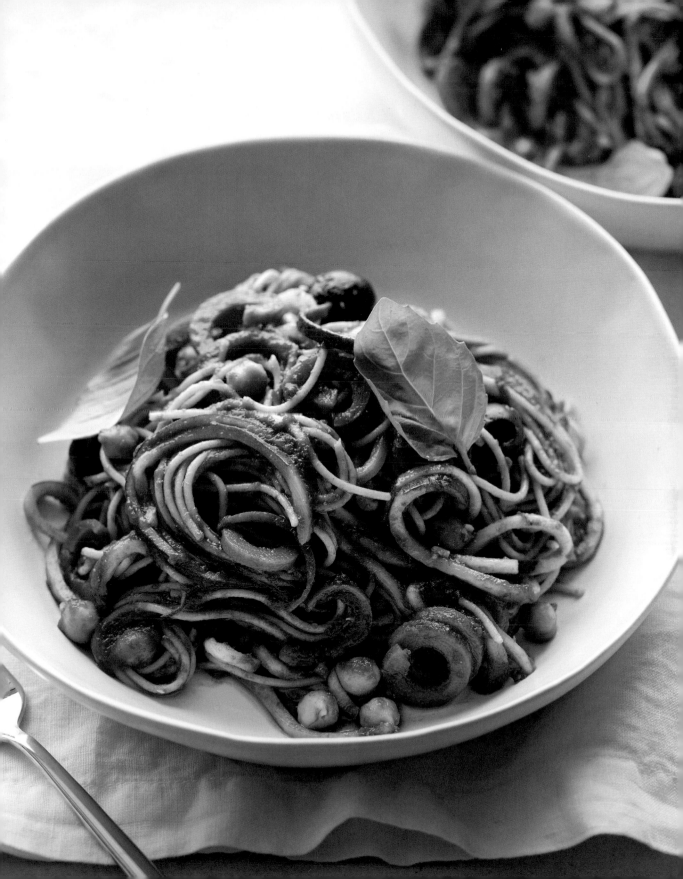

Lo Mein with Oyster Mushrooms and Chinese Broccoli

Makes about
6 cups

Ready in
25 minutes

Lo mein is a dish of Chinese noodles stir-fried with vegetables. Mine stays true to the original but without the greasiness you find in many restaurants. Chinese broccoli is similar to broccoli but with more leaves and smaller florets. You can find it in Asian grocery stores or use bok choy or broccolini in its place.

6 ounces long whole-grain noodles (such as spaghetti, Thai-style brown rice noodles, or soba or udon noodles)

1 tablespoon grated peeled fresh ginger

6 medium garlic cloves, minced (about 1 tablespoon)

¼ cup 30-Minute Vegetable Stock (page 32; or oil-free, low-sodium store-bought stock or water), plus more as needed

1 cup oyster mushrooms, trimmed (1 3-ounce package)

1 cup snow peas, cut diagonally into 1-inch pieces (about 1½ ounces)

1 medium red bell pepper, cored, seeded, and cut into thin strips (about 1 cup)

1 medium carrot, peeled and cut into matchsticks (about ¾ cup)

1 bunch Chinese broccoli (or ½ bunch broccolini), cut into 1-inch pieces,

including stems (about 1 cup)

2 tablespoons low-sodium tamari (or low-sodium soy sauce)

1 tablespoon rice wine vinegar

2 scallions, thinly sliced (white and green parts; about ½ cup)

1 teaspoon black or white toasted sesame seeds (optional)

1. Cook the noodles according to the package instructions. Drain in a colander and run cold water over them to stop them from cooking. Set aside.

2. Combine the ginger, garlic, and ¼ cup of the stock in a large sauté pan and cook over medium heat for 2 minutes. Add the mushrooms, snow peas, bell pepper, carrot, and broccoli and sauté for 5 to 7 minutes, until the vegetables are tender but not mushy, adding 1 to 2 more tablespoons of stock as needed to keep the vegetables from sticking to the pan. Add the noodles, tamari, and vinegar. Mix well and cook until the noodles are heated through. Garnish with the scallions and sesame seeds (if you're using them). Serve hot.

STORAGE: Refrigerate the noodles in an airtight container for up to 5 days.

Thai Noodle Salad with Mango-Lime Dressing

This noodle salad brings together the contrasting sweet and spicy flavors of Thai cuisine. I toss a lot of crunchy vegetables and fresh herbs into the mix, so it's really fresh and vibrant. The dressing is sweet, with some spiciness from the fresh ginger and cayenne pepper.

Makes about
9 cups

Ready in
25 minutes

For the Salad

6 ounces Thai-style brown rice noodles (or any whole-grain noodles, such as soba or udon noodles, or whole grain pasta)

4 medium carrots (about 6 ounces), peeled and grated on the large holes of a box grater (about 2 cups)

2 medium red bell peppers, cored, seeded, and cut into ½-inch dice (about 2 cups)

2 baby bok choy (about 12 ounces), cut into 1-inch dice (about 4 cups)

2 cups bean sprouts (about 4 ounces)

2 scallions, finely chopped (white and green parts; about ½ cup)

2 tablespoons finely chopped fresh mint

1 tablespoon roasted peanuts, crushed or coarsely chopped (optional)

For the Dressing

1½ cups chopped mango (fresh or frozen, thawed; about 12 ounces)

⅓ cup fresh lime juice

½ teaspoon grated peeled fresh ginger

2 tablespoons pure maple syrup

Pinch of cayenne pepper (optional)

Sea salt

1. To prepare the salad, cook the noodles according to the package instructions. Drain in a colander and run cold water over them to stop them from cooking. Transfer to a large bowl and set aside.

2. Combine the carrots, bell peppers, and bok choy in a large sauté pan and sauté with water for 3 to 5 minutes, folding the vegetables with a big spoon so they cook evenly, until the bok choy is wilted and the carrots are slightly tender. Transfer to the bowl with the noodles and set aside to cool to room temperature. Add the bean sprouts, scallions, and mint.

3. To make the dressing, combine the mango, lime juice, ginger, maple syrup, and

cayenne pepper (if you're using it) in a blender and blend into a smooth paste. Add salt to taste.

4. Spoon three-fourths of the dressing over the salad and toss to combine the ingredients and coat with the dressing; add the remaining dressing if desired. Sprinkle with the roasted peanuts (if you're using them). Serve at room temperature or chilled.

STORAGE: Refrigerate in an airtight container for up to 3 days.

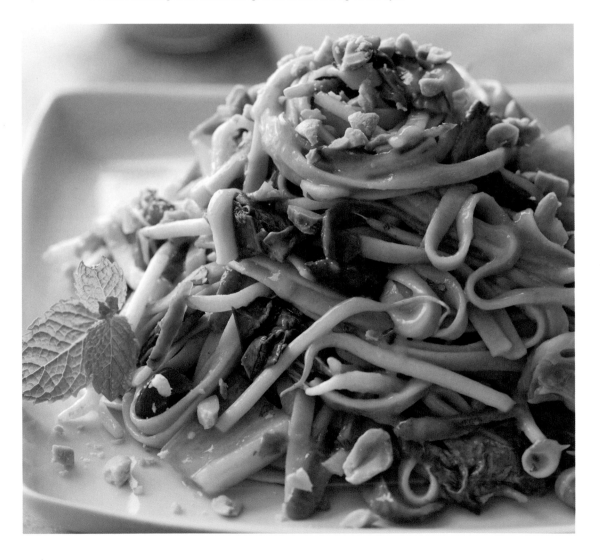

Potato Spaetzle with Green Peas and Shallot

I was introduced to spaetzle, a dish of knot-shaped egg noodles and sauce, while traveling in Germany years ago. The dish was so good that I wanted to re-create it, adapted to my whole-food, plant-based way of eating. When I did, it was even more delicious than the original because I added potatoes to the noodles, giving them more flavor. I toss the spaetzle with peas, which provide welcome little bursts of flavor. For a richer, heartier dish, top the spaetzle with French Lentil Ragout (page 191) or Myrna's Marinara Sauce (page 34).

Makes about
6 cups spaetzle

Ready in
45 minutes

1 shallot, cut into ¼-inch dice (about ½ cup)

1 cup fresh or frozen green peas (about 5 ounces)

1 pound Yukon Gold potatoes, peeled and cut into large pieces (about 4 cups)

1 cup whole-wheat flour

¼ teaspoon grated nutmeg

2 tablespoons finely chopped fresh parsley

Sea salt

Freshly ground black pepper

2 cups French Lentil Ragout (page 191; optional) or Myrna's Marinara Sauce (page 34; optional)

1. Sauté the shallot with ¼ cup water in a large sauté pan over medium heat for about 10 minutes, until it is soft, adding 1 to 2 more tablespoons of water as necessary to keep it from sticking to the pan. Add the peas and cook for another 5 minutes. Set aside.

2. Place a steamer basket in a medium saucepan and add 1 to 2 inches of water to the pan. Bring the water to a simmer over medium-high heat. Place the potatoes in the steamer, cover, and steam until tender when pierced with a fork, 5 to 7 minutes. Transfer the potatoes to a large bowl and mash them with a potato masher. Add the flour and nutmeg to the bowl with the potatoes. Using your hands, massage the mixture until the dough comes together.

3. Pinch the dough off in small clumps and roll the clumps into ¼-inch-thick strips. Using a dough scraper or a knife, cut the dough into 2-inch-long strips.

4. Bring a large pot of water to a boil over high heat. Drop half of the spaetzle into the water and cook them until they float to the top, about 20 seconds. Remove the spaetzle from the water and add them to the pot with the shallot and peas. Cook the remaining spaetzle in the same way and continue adding them to the pan with the shallot and peas.

5. Add the parsley and salt and pepper to taste and stir gently to distribute the seasonings without breaking up the spaetzle.

6. To serve, spoon the spaetzle into individual serving bowls. Spoon the lentils or marinara sauce on top, if you're using it.

STORAGE: Refrigerate the spaetzle (plain or tossed with the other ingredients) in an airtight container for up to 3 days or freeze for up to 1 month.

Soba Noodles with Shiitake Mushrooms and Eggplant

If you like spicy Asian food, you will love this noodle dish. The flavors come from the sautéed vegetables spiked with togarashi, a Japanese blend of chiles, nori, sesame seeds, and orange peel. I stumbled upon togarashi in an Asian supermarket. I tried it and liked it. Now I often add it to soups, cooked vegetables, salads, and noodle dishes. One of the nice things about this dish is that it can be served warm, at room temperature, or chilled.

Makes about
8 cups

Ready in
30 minutes

NOTE: Mirin is a rice wine with a low alcohol level that is commonly used in Japanese cooking. Yuzu is an Asian citrus fruit, the juice and rind of which are used in Japanese and Korean cuisine. I like to use these condiments to bring some authentic flavors to Japanese-themed recipes, but I find that brown rice vinegar and lemon zest make good substitutes without compromising much flavor.

6 ounces soba noodles (or udon noodles)

1 small onion, cut into ¼ inch dice (about 1 cup)

1 tablespoon grated peeled fresh ginger

6 medium garlic cloves, minced (about 1 tablespoon)

6 ounces shiitake mushrooms (or maitake mushrooms), trimmed and sliced ¼ inch thick (about 2 cups)

1 pound eggplant, peeled and cut into ½-inch-wide, 2-inch-long batons (about 4 Japanese eggplants or 2 small conventional eggplants)

1 cup jarred roasted red bell peppers, sliced (about 2 peppers)

3 tablespoons low-sodium tamari (or low-sodium soy sauce)

3 tablespoons mirin (or brown rice vinegar)

3 tablespoons yuzu juice (or fresh lemon juice)

12 cups fresh spinach (about 12 ounces)

2 tablespoons toasted sesame seeds (black or white or a mix)

Togarashi (or red pepper flakes)

1. Cook the noodles according to the package instructions. Reserve 1½ cups of the cooking water, drain the noodles in a colander, and run cold water over them to stop them from cooking. Set aside.

2. Combine the onion, ginger, and garlic in a large sauté pan and cook over medium heat for about 10 minutes, stirring occasionally, until the onion is golden brown, adding as little water as possible to keep the vegetables from sticking to the pan. (Too much water will keep the onion from browning; too little, and the ingredients will stick to the pan and burn.) Add the mushrooms, eggplant, bell peppers, tamari, mirin, and yuzu juice. Cover and cook for 5 to 7 minutes, until the eggplant is tender. Uncover.

3. If the noodles are stuck together, transfer them to a bowl and add ½ cup of the reserved pasta water. Gently toss with the water to untangle the noodles. Add the noodles, spinach, and 1 cup of the pasta water to the pan with the vegetables and toss to coat the noodles with the sauce in the pan. Sprinkle with the sesame seeds and togarashi or red pepper flakes. Serve warm, at room temperature, or chilled.

STORAGE: Refrigerate in an airtight container for up to 3 days.

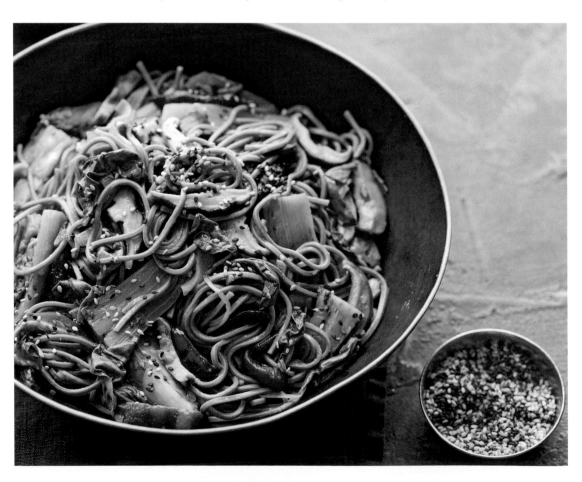

Khow Suey: Burmese Yellow Curry Noodles

Burmese cuisine has a lot of influences from its neighbors, including Thailand and my native India, so it feels both exotic and familiar to me. This brothy dish is a one-pot meal of noodles, vegetables, and curried soup. I've skipped the traditional coconut milk and thickened the soup instead with chickpea flour, which gives the soup a creamy texture without the fat of coconut milk.

Makes about 8 cups

Ready in 25 minutes

6 ounces long whole-grain noodles (such as spaghetti, Thai-style brown rice noodles, or soba or udon noodles)

½ small yellow onion, cut into ¼-inch dice (about ½ cup)

1½ tablespoons curry powder

4 medium garlic cloves, minced (about 2 teaspoons)

½ tablespoon grated peeled fresh ginger

3 tablespoons chickpea flour

4 cups fresh or frozen stir-fry vegetables (about 1 pound)

2 cups unsweetened, unflavored plant milk

Sea salt

2 scallions, thinly sliced (white and green parts; about ½ cup)

2 tablespoons finely chopped fresh cilantro, plus more for garnish

3 limes, cut into wedges

Sriracha (or another hot sauce) for serving

1. Cook the noodles according to the package instructions. Drain in a colander and run cold water over them to stop them from cooking. Set aside.

2. Combine the onion, curry powder, garlic, and ginger in a large saucepan or soup pot. Add ¼ cup water and sauté over medium-low heat for about 10 minutes, stirring occasionally, until the onion is tender.

3. In a small bowl, whisk the flour with 1 cup water until no lumps remain. Add this mixture, along with 1 cup water, to the pan with the onion mixture. Add the stir-fry vegetables and bring the liquid to a boil over high heat, stirring constantly. Reduce the heat to medium-low and simmer for about 10 minutes, until the vegetables are tender. Add the noodles and milk and cook for 3 to 4 minutes, until the noodles are warmed through. Add salt to taste.

4. Serve warm, garnished with the scallions and cilantro and with the lime wedges and sriracha on the side.

STORAGE: Refrigerate in an airtight container for up to 5 days or freeze for up to 1 month.

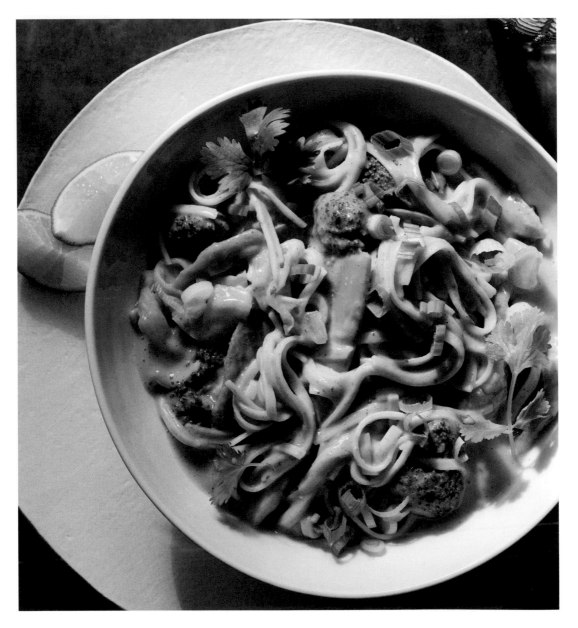

Forks Over Knives: Flavor!

Pasta Salad with Mixed Veggies and Corn-Basil Cream

I served this simple pasta salad at an office party not long ago, and it was a huge hit. It's my version of a classic American pasta salad, the type you might see at a picnic. The pasta is tossed with a creamy corn-basil sauce—the highlight of the dish—that provides a special flair and taste.

Makes about 6 cups

Ready in 15 minutes, plus 1 hour to chill

6 ounces whole-grain macaroni (about 1½ cups)

1½ cups frozen mixed small vegetables (such as peas, corn, and carrots; about 6 ounces)

2 celery stalks, cut into ¼-inch dice (about 1 cup)

⅛ red onion, minced

1 tablespoon white wine vinegar

1 cup Corn-Basil Cream (recipe follows)

Sea salt

Freshly ground black pepper

1. Cook the pasta according to the package instructions. During the last 5 minutes of cooking, add the frozen vegetables to the water with the pasta and cook for 5 minutes. Reserve 1 cup of the cooking water, drain the pasta and vegetables in a colander, and run cold water over them to stop them from cooking. Set aside to cool to room temperature.

2. Transfer the pasta and vegetables to a large bowl. Add the celery, onion, vinegar, and corn-basil cream and toss to coat the pasta and veggies with the dressing. Season with salt and pepper to taste. Cover and refrigerate for at least 1 hour before serving. Serve chilled.

STORAGE: Refrigerate in an airtight container for up to 3 days.

Corn-Basil Cream

Makes about 1 cup

Ready in
25 minutes

This basil-flavored sauce has a creamy texture and a pretty bright green color. I've made it with several varieties of fresh corn. Golden corn (as opposed to white corn) gives the best results, because it has a lot of flavor without being too sweet. That said, you can even use frozen corn kernels in a pinch. I use the sauce to toss the Pasta Salad with Mixed Veggies and Corn-Basil Cream (recipe above) and also as a dipping sauce for fresh vegetables.

3 cups fresh or frozen corn kernels (from about 3 large cobs)

1 tablespoon white wine vinegar

1 tablespoon fresh lemon juice

1 teaspoon yellow mustard

1 teaspoon garlic powder

1 packed cup fresh basil

Freshly ground black pepper

Black salt (optional)

1. Combine the corn with ½ cup water in a blender and puree.

2. Strain the puree through a fine mesh strainer into a large sauté pan. Add the vinegar, lemon juice, mustard, and garlic powder and bring to a boil over high heat. Reduce the heat to medium-low and simmer for 5 to 7 minutes, until the sauce thickens slightly. Turn off the heat and set aside to cool to room temperature.

3. Return the sauce to the blender, add the basil, and blend until the basil is finely chopped and the sauce is green. Add the pepper and black salt (if you're using it) to taste.

STORAGE: Refrigerate in an airtight container for up to 5 days.

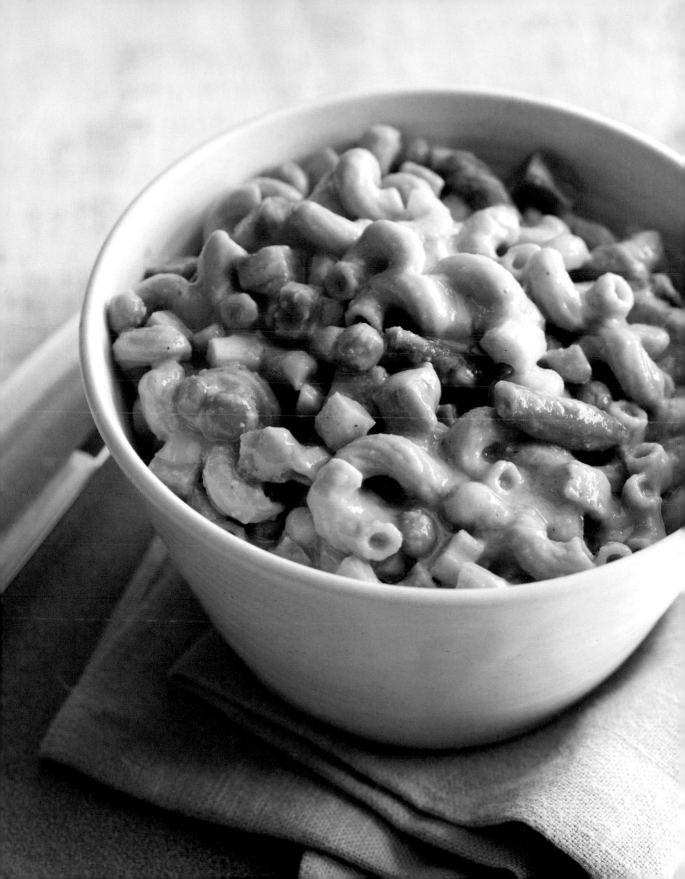

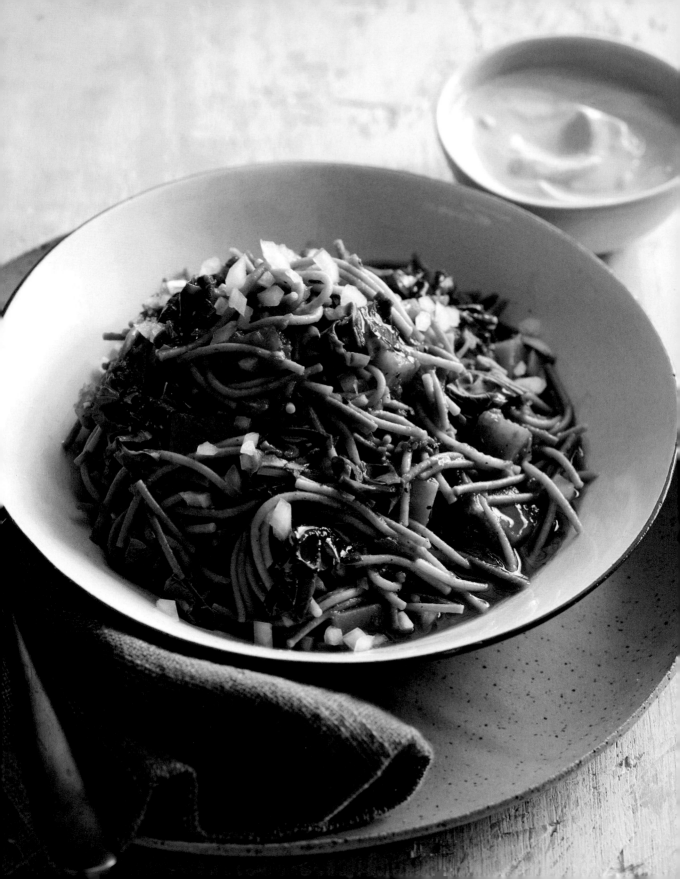

Sopa de Fideo: Mexican Noodle Casserole

Sopa de fideo is a hearty, tomato-based Mexican noodle dish. It can range from a traditional soup consistency to that of a baked noodle casserole. Here, I've made the casserole-like version, adding Swiss chard and butternut squash to turn it into a one-dish meal.

Makes about 10 cups

Ready in 30 minutes

NOTE: To make this into a traditional soupy consistency, add 3 additional cups of stock or water to the recipe.

1 medium yellow onion

1 (15-ounce) can sodium-free or low-sodium fire-roasted tomatoes (about 1½ cups)

4 medium garlic cloves

1 jalapeño pepper, seeded

4 ounces whole-grain spaghetti, broken into 2-inch segments (about 2 cups)

1 cup peeled (½-inch-diced) butternut squash (about 5 ounces)

½ bunch Swiss chard, stems removed and discarded, leaves shredded (about 2 cups)

1 tablespoon fresh lime juice

Sea salt

Chipotle "Sour Cream" (page 335) or Tofu "Sour Cream" (page 334)

1. Finely dice enough of the onion to get ¼ cup and cut the rest into big chunks.

2. Put the onion chunks into a blender. Add the tomatoes, garlic, and jalapeño. Fill the tomato can with water and add it to the blender. (Or simply add 1½ cups water.) Puree until smooth.

3. Toast the spaghetti in a large sauté pan over medium-high heat, stirring frequently so it does not burn, until it is deep golden and fragrant, about 6 minutes. Scatter the butternut squash over the pasta and pour the pureed sauce evenly over the top. Cover and cook over medium-low heat until the squash is tender, 15 to 20 minutes. Uncover, lay the chard on top, and return the lid to the pot. Cook for about 2 minutes to wilt the chard. Uncover and sprinkle with the lime juice and salt to taste.

4. To serve, drizzle with the "sour cream" and sprinkle the chopped onion on top. Serve warm.

STORAGE: Let the soup cool to room temperature and transfer it to a container with a tight-fitting lid. Refrigerate for up to 5 days.

Japanese Cold Noodle Salad with Citrus Dressing

Makes about 7 cups

Ready in
20 minutes

This is a simple salad of noodles and vegetables tossed with a refreshing dressing. I make the dressing with yuzu, a Japanese citrus fruit known for its sourness. You will find bottled yuzu juice in specialty or Japanese markets and fresh yuzu in some supermarkets. If you cannot find it, use lemon juice and a few gratings of lemon zest in its place.

¼ cup arame seaweed (or any other seaweed; optional)

6 ounces soba or udon noodles

6 cups fresh spinach (preferably baby spinach; about 6 ounces)

3 tablespoons Date Paste (page 30)

3 tablespoons brown rice vinegar

2 tablespoons yuzu juice (or fresh lemon juice mixed with several gratings of lemon rind)

1½ tablespoons mild white miso

1½ tablespoons grated peeled fresh ginger

2 medium carrots, peeled and grated (about 1 cup)

½ cup frozen edamame, thawed (about 5 ounces)

2 scallions, thinly sliced (white and green parts; about ½ cup)

1 tablespoon toasted sesame seeds (preferably black sesame seeds)

1. If you are using arame, soak it in a bowlful of water for 10 minutes to leach out some of the sodium. Bring a small pot of water to a boil over high heat. Drain the arame and add it to the boiling water. Reduce the heat to medium and simmer for 5 minutes. Drain and rinse the arame.

2. Cook the noodles according to the package instructions. While the noodles are still in the pot of water, add the spinach and cook for 15 seconds. Drain the noodles and spinach in a colander and run under cold water to stop them from cooking. Transfer the noodles and spinach to a large bowl.

3. Meanwhile, combine the date paste, vinegar, yuzu juice, miso, and ginger in a

small bowl to make the dressing. Use a fork to break up the miso and date paste and combine the ingredients.

4. Add the arame (if you're using it), carrots, edamame, scallions, sesame seeds, and dressing to the bowl with the noodles and toss to combine. Serve at room temperature or chilled.

STORAGE: Refrigerate in an airtight container for up to 5 days.

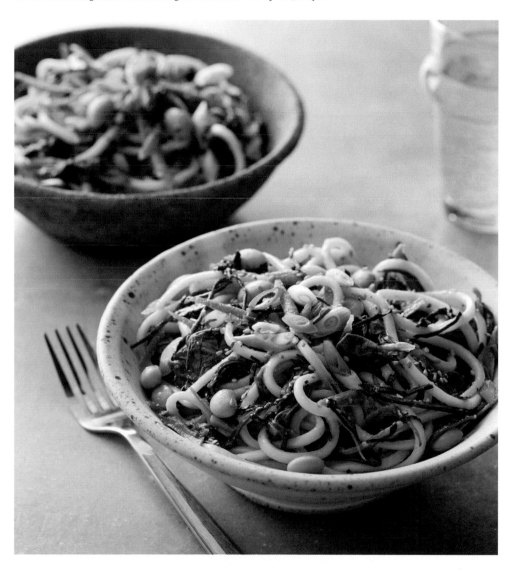

Whole grains and beans are the foundation of a healthy diet. Combined with vegetables, herbs, and other flavors, they turn into vibrant and delicious meals that can be served alongside bolder flavors, or enjoyed as stand-alone dishes.

9 | Grains and Beans

Bibimbap: Korean Rice Bowl

Bibimbap, which means "mixed rice," is a classic Korean bowl of rice topped with a selection of vegetables and meats, and served with a variety of condiments. Brian and I often order a vegan version at our favorite local Asian fusion restaurant; the chef there is nice enough to make ours oil-free. This recipe, which includes vegetables that are raw, cooked, and pickled, makes for a delightful mix of colors, textures, and flavors.

½ (12- to 16-ounce) package extra-firm tofu

2 cups wild mushrooms (such as enoki, shiitake, wood ear, or a combination; about 3½ ounces), trimmed and thinly sliced

1 teaspoon grated peeled fresh ginger

2 medium garlic cloves, minced (about 1 teaspoon)

1 tablespoon low-sodium tamari (or low-sodium soy sauce)

2 cups fresh spinach (about 2 ounces), finely chopped

1 cup (¾-inch cubed) acorn squash (about one-fourth of a squash)

2 cups bean sprouts (about 4 ounces)

For Serving

3 cups cooked brown rice (from 1 cup uncooked rice)

2 scallions, thinly sliced (white and green parts; about ½ cup)

Gochujang (page 343; or sriracha)

Quick Vegetable Pickle (page 82)

1. Drain the tofu and press it between your hands to remove excess liquid. Cut the tofu into 1-inch cubes. Heat a large nonstick sauté pan over medium heat for 2 minutes. Add the tofu cubes and cook until they are golden brown on all sides, about 5 minutes, turning them so they brown evenly. Remove the tofu from the sauté pan and set aside.

2. In the same sauté pan you used to cook the tofu, sauté the mushrooms, ginger, and garlic over medium-high heat for about 5 minutes, stirring occasionally, until the mushrooms are tender. Add the tofu to the sauté pan. Drizzle with the tamari, and toss gently to combine. Transfer to a bowl and set aside in a warm place.

3. Add the spinach to the sauté pan you cooked the tofu and mushrooms in (no need to wipe out the pan) and sauté for 3 to 5 minutes, until wilted.

4. Meanwhile, place a steamer basket in a medium saucepan and add 1 to 2 inches of water to the pan. Bring the water to a simmer over medium-high heat. Place the squash in the steamer, cover, and steam until barely tender when pierced with a fork, about 7 minutes. Add the bean sprouts and steam for 3 minutes. Uncover and remove the vegetables from the steamer.

5. To serve, spoon the rice into individual bowls. Pile the tofu, sautéed vegetables, steamed vegetables, and pickled vegetables in separate mounds on top of the rice. Garnish with the scallions and serve with the gochujang and quick vegetable pickle on the side.

STORAGE: Refrigerate the various components in separate covered containers for up to 4 days.

"You do not need to add water when sautéeing mushrooms. They release a lot of water as they cook; adding water will give them an unpleasantly spongy texture."

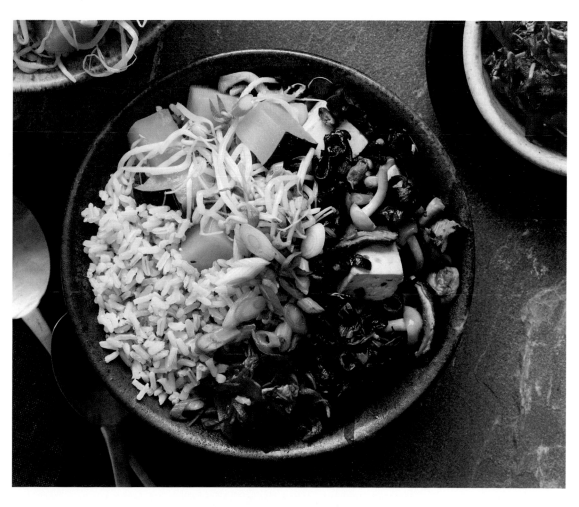

Multigrain Grits with Succotash

Makes about
6 cups

Ready in
45 minutes

Grits, a savory porridgelike side dish made from coarsely ground cornmeal, are a staple of Southern cuisine. They are basically the American version of Italian polenta, which is a real comfort food for me. I use a combination of cornmeal, amaranth, and millet to make the grits, which gives the dish different nuances of flavor. Succotash, a vegetable dish of corn and lima beans, is often served with grits. In this recipe, I add oyster mushrooms to the mix to give it an umami flavor.

For the Grits

2 cups unsweetened, unflavored plant milk, plus more as needed

⅓ cup cornmeal

⅓ cup amaranth

⅓ cup millet, rinsed and drained

1 tablespoon nutritional yeast

For the Succotash

1 cup frozen lima beans (about 5 ounces)

1 small yellow onion, cut into ¼-inch dice (about ½ cup)

3 medium garlic cloves, minced (about ½ tablespoon)

2 cups oyster mushrooms, trimmed (4 to 5 ounces), cut into 1-inch pieces

1½ cups fresh or frozen corn kernels (from about 1½ large cobs)

1 small tomato (about 4 ounces), cut into ½-inch dice

1 teaspoon white wine vinegar

Sea salt

Freshly ground black pepper

1 tablespoon finely chopped fresh parsley

1. To make the grits, combine the milk with 2 cups water in a medium saucepan and bring to a boil over high heat. Add the cornmeal, amaranth, millet, and nutritional yeast and stir to combine. Reduce the heat to medium-low, cover, and simmer for 25 to 30 minutes, until the grains are tender and the liquid is absorbed. Turn off the heat and set aside.

2. Meanwhile, to make the succotash, combine the lima beans, onion, and garlic in a large sauté pan. Add ¼ cup water and cook over medium heat for about 10 minutes, until the onion is tender, adding 1 to 2 more tablespoons of water as needed to keep the vegetables from sticking to the pan. Add the mushrooms, corn, to-

mato, vinegar, and salt and pepper to taste and cook for 5 to 7 minutes, until the mushrooms are tender. Turn off the heat and stir in the parsley.

3. To serve, if the grits have cooled, warm them over medium-low heat, adding more plant milk or water as necessary to achieve a loose, spoonable consistency. Spoon the grits into individual bowls and top with the succotash.

STORAGE: Refrigerate the grits and succotash in separate covered containers for up to 4 days. Reheat the grits over medium-low heat, adding more plant milk or water as necessary.

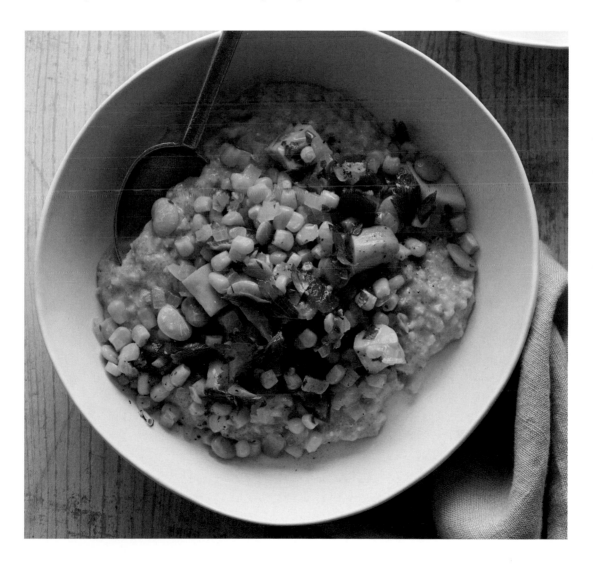

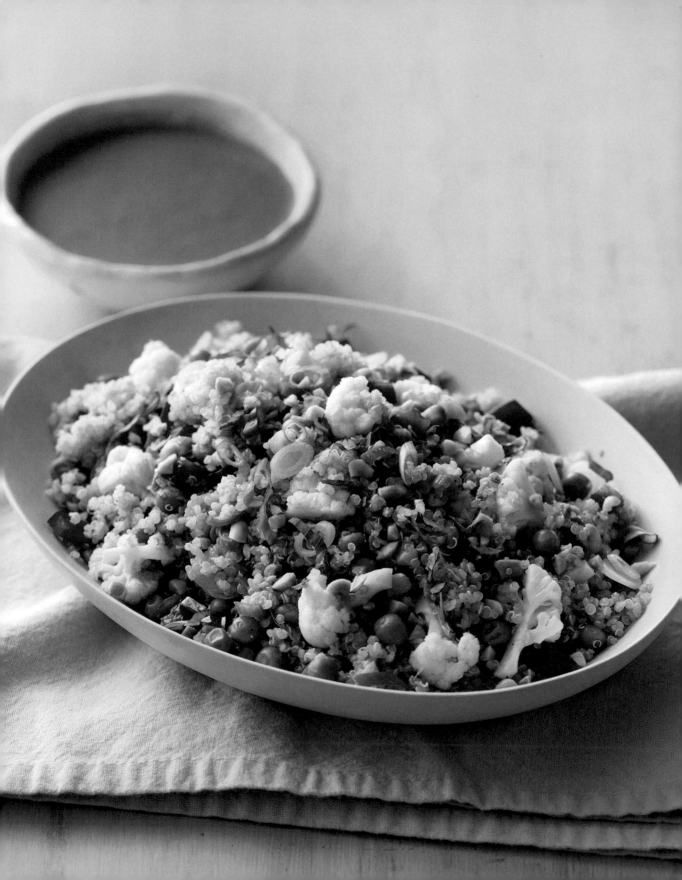

Thai Quinoa Salad with Peanut Sauce

This quinoa salad or side dish is easy to make, yet it has all the complexity of flavor that is the signature of Thai cuisine. I serve it with Thai Green Curry with Lima Beans (page 218) or on its own, with Peanut Sauce (page 337) drizzled on top. The quinoa salad is a great dish to take to a picnic or to work because it stays fresh throughout the day.

Makes about 6 cups

Ready in 30 minutes

1 cup quinoa, rinsed and drained

2 tablespoons Thai Green Curry Paste (page 219) (or Thai Red Curry Paste, page 251, or store-bought curry paste)

2 medium garlic cloves, minced (about 1 teaspoon)

1 teaspoon grated peeled fresh ginger

1 medium red bell pepper, cored, seeded, and cut into ¼-inch dice (about 1 cup)

1 cup (¼-inch) cauliflower florets

1 cup fresh or frozen green peas (about 5 ounces)

¼ cup fresh lemon juice

3 scallions, thinly sliced (white and green parts; about ¾ cup)

¼ cup thinly sliced fresh basil (preferably Thai basil)

2 tablespoons crushed roasted peanuts

Sea salt

Freshly ground black pepper

Peanut Sauce (page 337)

1. Put the quinoa into a medium saucepan and dry toast it over medium low-heat for 5 minutes, shaking the pan occasionally. Add the curry paste, garlic, ginger, and 2 cups water and bring to a boil over high heat. Reduce the heat to medium-low, cover, and simmer for 15 to 18 minutes, until no liquid remains.

2. Uncover the pot and scatter the bell pepper, cauliflower, and peas evenly over the quinoa. Sprinkle with the lemon juice, cover the pot, and let stand for 10 minutes. Uncover the pot. Add the scallions, basil, peanuts, and salt and pepper to taste and use a fork to fluff up the quinoa and combine the ingredients. Serve warm or chilled with the peanut sauce on the side.

STORAGE: Refrigerate in an airtight container for up to 4 days.

Paella de Verduras

Makes about
10 cups

Ready in 1 hour

With its colorful presentation and variety of ingredients, paella feels like a special-occasion dish. As a cook, one of the things I appreciate about paella is how many different ways I can prepare it. The butter beans and trumpet mushrooms in this recipe give this one a hearty, distinct flavor and add a satisfying, chewy texture to the rice-based dish.

1 cup short-grain (or long-grain) brown rice, rinsed and drained

½ pound trumpet mushrooms (or any mushrooms), trimmed and cut into ¾-inch dice (about 3 cups)

1 medium yellow onion, cut into ¼-inch dice (about 2 cups)

3 medium garlic cloves, minced (about 1½ teaspoons)

1 (15-ounce) can sodium-free or low-sodium diced tomatoes, drained (about 1 cup)

1 medium red bell pepper, cored, seeded, and cut into ¼-inch dice (about 1 cup)

1 tablespoon smoked paprika

1 teaspoon dried parsley

¼ teaspoon cayenne pepper

½ teaspoon sea salt

⅛ teaspoon saffron threads

6 ounces green beans, cut into 1½-inch segments (about 1 cup)

1 cup (1-inch) broccoli florets (from 1 small head broccoli)

1 medium yellow zucchini (or any summer squash), cut into ½-inch dice (about 1 cup)

1 (15-ounce) can butter beans (or lima beans), rinsed and drained (about 1½ cups)

1 lemon, cut into 6 wedges

1. Soak the rice in 2 cups hot water for 20 minutes. Drain and rinse.

2. In a wide, straight-sided sauté pan or Dutch oven, combine the mushrooms, onion, and garlic and sauté over medium heat for about 10 minutes, stirring occasionally, until the onion is tender; you won't need to add any water while cooking, as the mushrooms will release enough water to keep the vegetables from sticking to the pan or burning.

3. Add the rice, tomatoes, bell pepper, paprika, parsley, cayenne pepper, salt, and saffron to the pot with the mushrooms and onion. Stir to combine the ingredients and

cook for 5 to 7 minutes to toast the spices and soften the bell pepper. Add 2 cups water and bring to a boil over high heat. Reduce the heat to medium-low, cover, and simmer for about 50 minutes, until the rice is tender and the liquid is absorbed.

4. Meanwhile, place a steamer basket in a medium saucepan, add 1 to 2 inches of water to the pan, and bring the water to a simmer over medium-high heat. Place the green beans in the steamer, cover, and steam for 5 minutes. Uncover, add the broccoli and zucchini to the steamer, cover again, and steam for 5 minutes. Uncover.

5. Transfer the vegetables to the pot with the rice. Add the butter beans and mix to combine. Cover and let stand for 10 minutes. Serve warm with the lemon wedges on the side.

STORAGE: Refrigerate in an airtight container for up to 4 days.

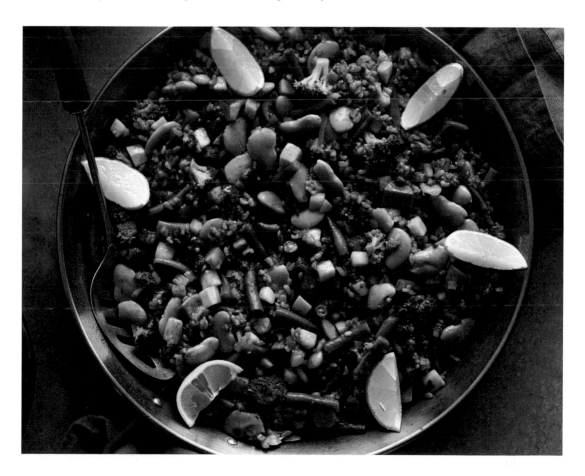

Mushroom and Kale Farrotto

Makes about 5 cups

Ready in
40 minutes

Farrotto is like risotto but made from farro, an ancient Italian grain in the wheat family, rather than rice. Mushrooms and kale make this version rich and hearty, perfect for a cold night.

1 cup farro, rinsed and drained

2 cups 30-Minute Vegetable Stock (page 32; or oil-free, low-sodium store-bought stock or water)

1 medium yellow onion, cut into ¼-inch dice (about 2 cups)

4 ounces mushrooms (any variety or a combination), trimmed and thinly sliced (about 1½ cups)

6 medium garlic cloves, minced (about 1 tablespoon)

1 cup unsweetened, unflavored plant milk, plus more as needed

2 tablespoons tomato paste

½ bunch kale, stems removed and discarded, leaves finely chopped (about 2 cups)

1 teaspoon white wine vinegar

1 tablespoon finely chopped fresh oregano

Sea salt

Freshly ground black pepper

Frozen Cashew Chickpea "Cheese" (page 35) or nutritional yeast

1. Combine the farro and stock in a medium saucepan and bring to a boil over high heat. Cover the pot, reduce the heat to medium-low, and simmer for 20 minutes to partially cook the farro. Drain off the excess stock and reserve.

2. Combine the onion, mushrooms, and garlic in a separate large saucepan and sauté over medium heat for about 10 minutes, until the onion is tender and translucent, stirring frequently and adding 1 to 2 tablespoons of the reserved stock or water as needed to keep the vegetables from sticking to the pan. Add the farro, milk, tomato paste, kale, vinegar, oregano, and salt and pepper to taste and cook over medium heat, stirring frequently, for 10 to 15 minutes, until the grains are tender and the farrotto has a creamy texture; add more milk or water if necessary for the farrotto to achieve a loose, spoonable consistency.

3. To serve, spoon the farrotto into individual bowls and grate the "cheese" or sprinkle the nutritional yeast over it. Serve warm.

STORAGE: Refrigerate in an airtight container for up to 4 days. Reheat over medium-low heat, adding water to the pan to loosen the farrotto to a spoonable, creamy consistency.

Coconut Ginger Red Rice

Brian and I recently took a trip to Sri Lanka. I fell in love with a rice preparation that I had there, where the rice was cooked with freshly grated coconut. When I replicated the dish back home, I lightened it up by adding shredded jicama in place of some of the coconut. This rice makes a good accompaniment to any soup, stew, or curry.

Makes about
4 cups

Ready in
45 minutes

NOTE: Sri Lankan cuisine uses a few different varieties of red rice, none of which is available here, so I use Thai red rice instead. It has a nutty flavor that goes well with the coconut and a pretty pink color. If you can't find red rice, use long-grain brown rice instead. Curry leaves are an ingredient unique to South Asian cuisine. They are not something that is usually sold dried, like, for instance, bay leaves. You can buy fresh curry leaves at Indian and some Middle Eastern grocery stores. Freeze fresh curry leaves in a sealed plastic bag. If you can't find them, skip them, as there is no substitute.

1 teaspoon black mustard seeds	1 tablespoon grated peeled fresh ginger	2 tablespoons shredded coconut
½ medium yellow onion, cut into ¼-inch dice (about 1 cup)	1 sprig of curry leaves (4 to 6 leaves; optional)	2 tablespoons finely chopped fresh cilantro
6 medium garlic cloves, minced (about 1 tablespoon)	¼ jicama, peeled and grated on the large holes of a box grater (about 1 cup)	1 tablespoon fresh lime juice
	1½ cups Thai red rice (or long-grain brown rice), rinsed and drained	Sea salt

1. Toast the mustard seeds in a small, dry sauté pan over medium-low heat, shaking often, for 3 to 5 minutes, until they start to pop. Add the onion, garlic, ginger, curry leaves (if you're using them), and ¼ cup water and cook for 5 minutes. Add the jicama, rice, and 3 cups water and bring to a boil over high heat. Reduce the heat to medium-low, cover, and simmer for 30 to 40 minutes, until the liquid is absorbed. Turn off the heat and let the rice rest, covered, for 10 minutes.

2. Uncover and add the coconut, cilantro, lime juice, and salt to taste and fluff with a fork to distribute the ingredients.

3. Serve warm with a stew, soup, curry, or stir-fry.

STORAGE: Refrigerate in an airtight container for up to 4 days.

Persian Dill and Lima Bean Pilaf

Makes about
8 cups

Ready in
40 minutes

Called *baghali polo* in Persian, this is one of the most popular rice dishes in Persian cuisine. It is incredibly fragrant with fresh dill and saffron. I sometimes make it with millet or quinoa instead of rice, just to mix things up a bit. It makes a perfect side for Persian Yellow Split Pea and Eggplant Stew (page 197).

NOTE: I use finely chopped lemon rind in this. It has a different effect from rind that is grated; with finely chopped rind, you get some of the white of the rind, not just the outer layer. I do this in place of using dried lemon rind, which would traditionally be added to this rice dish. It has a similar flavor and prevents you from having to seek out the dried product at a Middle Eastern specialty market. If you do find yourself at such a specialty market and can buy dried lemon rind, use that instead.

3 pinches saffron

1½ medium yellow onions, cut into ¼-inch dice (about 3 cups)

6 medium garlic cloves, minced (about 1 tablespoon)

1 tablespoon finely chopped fresh lemon rind (from about 1 lemon; or 1 whole dried lemon)

6 cups cooked brown basmati rice (from 1½ cups uncooked rice)

1½ cups frozen lima beans

¾ cup finely chopped fresh dill

3 tablespoons fresh lemon juice

Sea salt

Freshly ground black pepper

1. Mix the saffron with 2 tablespoons hot water in a small bowl.

2. Combine the onion, garlic, lemon rind (or dried lemon), and ¼ cup water in a large sauté pan and cook over medium heat for 10 minutes. Add the rice, beans, dill, lemon juice, and salt and pepper to taste and stir to combine. Drizzle the saffron water evenly over the pan. Cover and cook over low heat for 10 to 15 minutes, until the rice and beans are warmed through.

3. Uncover and fluff gently with a fork. (If you used a whole dried lemon, remove and discard it.) Serve with Persian Yellow Split Pea and Eggplant Stew (page 197).

STORAGE: Refrigerate in an airtight container for up to 4 days.

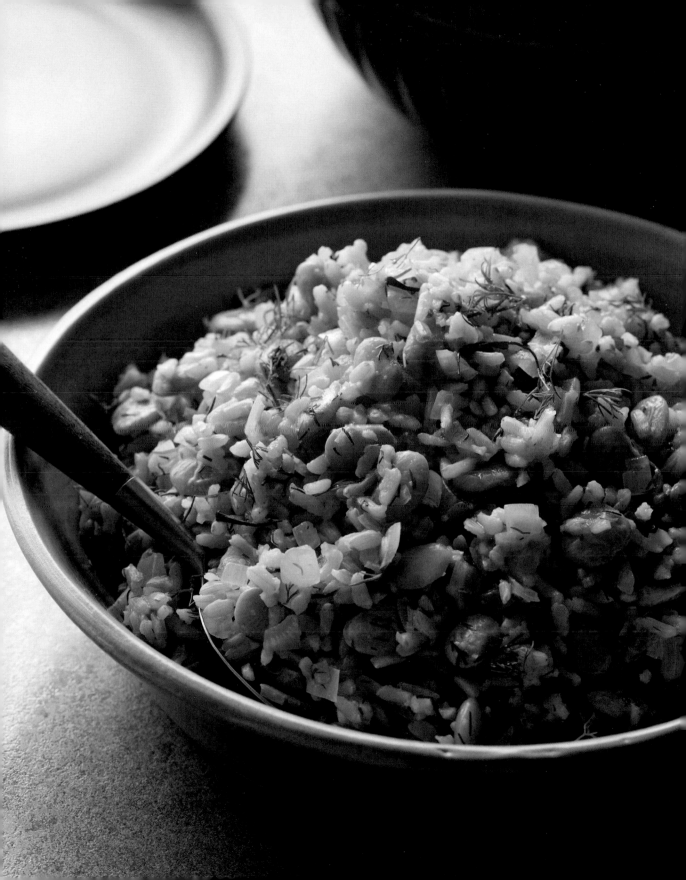

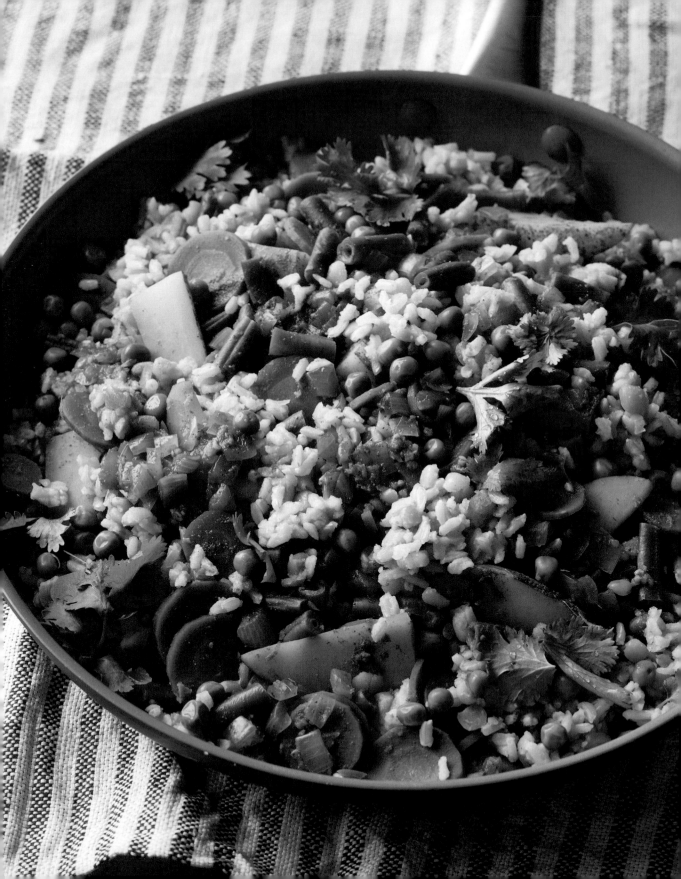

Royal Khichri

Khichri is a staple Indian dish of rice and lentils cooked together. It can be made into a dry pilaf-type dish or have a wetter, porridgelike texture; this one is more pilaflike. Each region of India has its own version of khichri, and within the regions, each family has its own recipe. My mom has many recipes for khichri, but this is the most popular in our family. It is called *badshahi khichri*, or "fit for the king." I named this dish Royal Khichri, even though I simplified Mom's recipe. Khichri is great for feeding a large crowd.

Makes about
9 cups

Ready in 1 hour

NOTE: This recipe uses yellow lentils, which are also known as yellow pigeon peas or toor dal. These legumes are available in most Indian or Persian markets and online. I suggest you seek them out rather than substituting another variety of peas or lentils, because the cooking time for them is the same as that for brown rice and they are cooked together in this recipe.

For the Khichri
¾ cup brown basmati rice (uncooked)

¾ cup yellow lentils (also known as toor dal or yellow pigeon peas)

For the Vegetables
1 large yellow onion, cut into ¼-inch dice (about 3 cups)

9 medium garlic cloves, minced (about 1½ tablespoons)

1 tablespoon grated peeled fresh ginger

1 tablespoon ground coriander

1 tablespoon garam masala

1 teaspoon ground cumin

¼ teaspoon ground turmeric

¼ teaspoon ground nutmeg

1 medium russet potato (about ½ pound), cut into 2-inch-long wedges

6 ounces green beans, trimmed and cut into 1-inch pieces (about 1 cup)

2 medium carrots, peeled and thinly sliced into rings (about 1 cup)

½ cup fresh or frozen peas (about 2½ ounces)

2 tablespoons finely chopped fresh cilantro leaves and stems, plus more for garnish

2 tablespoons fresh lime juice

Sea salt

1. To make the khichri, combine the rice, lentils, and 3 cups water in a large saucepan and bring the water to a boil over high heat. Reduce the heat to medium-low, cover, and gently simmer for about 40 minutes, until the rice and legumes are tender.

2. Meanwhile, to make the vegetables, combine the onion, garlic, ginger, coriander, garam masala, cumin, turmeric, and nutmeg in a large Dutch oven (or another large pan with straight, high sides). Add 1 cup water, cover, and simmer over medium heat for about 10 minutes, until the onion is tender. Uncover and spread the potatoes, green beans, and carrots over the onion. Cover and cook the vegetables for about 15 minutes, adding 1 to 2 more tablespoons of water as needed to prevent the vegetables from sticking to the pan, until they are tender. Uncover the pan and stir in the peas, cilantro, lime juice, and salt to taste.

3. Spread the khichri (rice and yellow lentils mixture) over the vegetables, cover the pan, and cook over medium heat for 5 minutes, or until the rice and lentils are heated through. Turn off the heat and uncover the pan.

4. To serve, gently fold the vegetables and the khichri together, being careful not to mix them completely. (I like to keep patches of rice and patches of vegetables rather than stirring everything together completely; I think it looks better that way, and I also think it improves the texture of the dish.) Garnish with cilantro.

STORAGE: Refrigerate in an airtight container for up to 4 days.

Mujadara Bowls with Parsley Tahini Sauce

Mujadara is a Middle Eastern medley of lentils, rice, and caramelized onions. On a recent trip to Vancouver, Brian and I found a Middle Eastern restaurant where the mujadara was so good we ordered it three times in the same week, along with salad and hummus. I turned that winning combination into a bowl.

Makes about 4 cups

Ready in 40 minutes

For the Mujadara

1 medium yellow onion (about 8 ounces), thinly sliced

1 medium carrot, peeled and cut into ½-inch dice (about ½ cup)

1 large zucchini, cut into 1-inch-long, ½-inch-thick batons (about 1 cup)

2 medium tomatoes, cut into wedges

1 cup brown lentils

½ teaspoon ground cumin

1 cup bulgur wheat

1 tablespoon fresh lemon juice

Sea salt

Freshly ground black pepper

For the Bowls

2 cups chopped lettuce (any variety)

1 cup Parsley Tahini Sauce (page 341)

¼ cup Harissa (page 344; optional)

1. To make the mujadara, preheat the oven to 450°F. Line a baking sheet with parchment paper.

2. Lay the onion slices on one half of the prepared baking sheet and the carrot, zucchini, and tomatoes on the other half. Bake in the oven for 15 minutes. Remove from the oven and gently stir the vegetables, keeping the onion slices separate from the other vegetables. Return the sheet to the oven and bake for 15 to 20 minutes, until the vegetables brown around the edges. Remove from the oven.

3. Bring 3 cups water to a boil in a medium saucepan over high heat. Add the lentils and cumin. Reduce the heat to medium, cover, and simmer for about 20 minutes, until the lentils are tender. Turn off the heat. Uncover and stir in the bulgur. Cover and set aside for 10 minutes to steam the grains.

4. Uncover, add the caramelized onion and lemon juice, and season with salt and pepper to taste. Fluff with a fork to combine the ingredients.

5. To serve, spoon the mujadara into individual bowls. Arrange the roasted vegetables and chopped lettuce on top and serve with the parsley tahini sauce and harissa (if you are using it) on the side.

STORAGE: Refrigerate in an airtight container for up to 3 days.

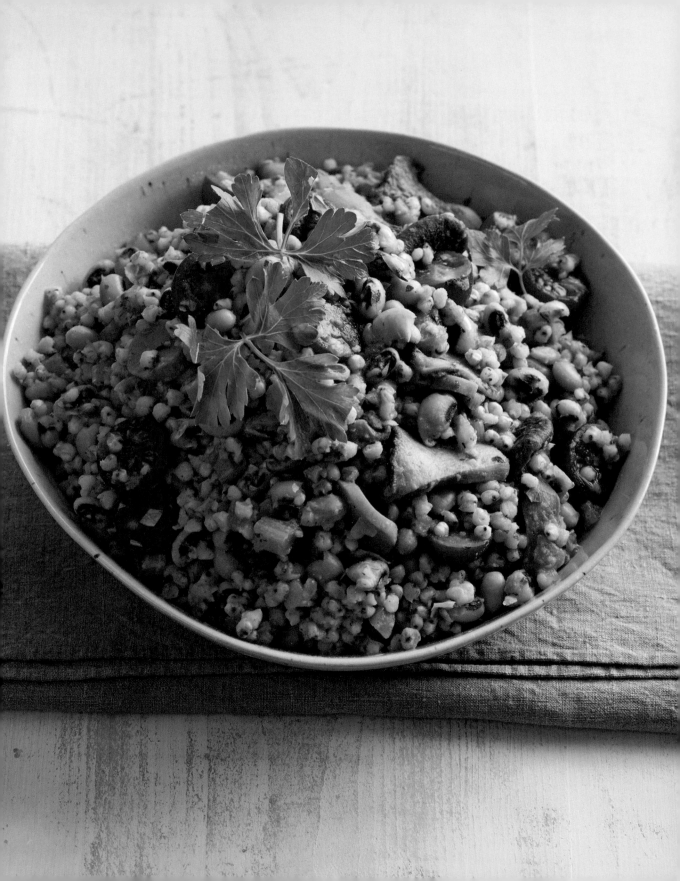

Sorghum Hoppin' John

This recipe is loosely based on the classic Southern Hoppin' John, a black-eyed pea and rice dish that includes bacon, onion, and spices. It is often served on New Year's Day, because it is thought to bring about good luck. In this vegan version, I combine the peas with sorghum instead of rice because I like its chewy, hearty quality. I cook the peas and the sorghum separately so the sorghum keeps its pretty, creamy color.

Makes about 7 cups

Ready in 1 hour,
10 minutes

1 cup sorghum, rinsed and drained

1 medium yellow onion, cut into ¼-inch dice (about 2 cups)

4 celery stalks, cut into ¼-inch dice (about 1½ cups)

9 medium garlic cloves, minced (about 1½ tablespoons)

2 teaspoons Italian seasoning

6 ounces trumpet mushrooms (or other wild mushrooms), trimmed and cut into ¼-inch slices (about 2 cups)

1 cup dried black-eyed peas

2 dried bay leaves

1 cup cherry tomatoes (about 6 ounces), cut in half

2 tablespoons red wine vinegar

Sea salt

Freshly ground black pepper

2 tablespoons finely chopped fresh parsley

1. Combine the sorghum and 2½ cups water in a medium saucepan and bring to a boil over high heat. Reduce the heat to medium-low, cover the pot, and simmer for 60 to 90 minutes, until the sorghum is tender.

2. Combine the onion, celery, garlic, and Italian seasoning in a large sauté pan and cook for about 10 minutes over medium heat until the vegetables are tender, adding ¼ cup water to keep the vegetables from sticking to the pan. Add the mushrooms, peas, bay leaves, and 2½ cups water and bring to a boil over high heat. Reduce the heat to medium-low and simmer for 45 minutes to 1 hour, until the beans are tender and the liquid is absorbed. (The time will vary depending on the freshness of the beans.)

3. Add the sorghum, tomatoes, and vinegar to the pan with the beans and vegetables. Mix well and add salt and pepper to taste. Cover and let stand for 10 minutes. Remove and discard the bay leaves and serve warm, garnished with the parsley.

STORAGE: Refrigerate in an airtight container for up to 3 days.

Mexican Rice with Poblano Chile and Creamed Corn

Makes about
4 cups

Ready in 1 hour

Many Mexican rice dishes are red in color from tomatoes. I decided to go a different direction and use pureed corn to give the rice a creamy texture and a sweet corn flavor. I love it with Sweet Potato Tortilla Soup (page 184) or any dish with a south-of-the-border flavor. I also like this rice on its own as a simple, flavorful lunch or snack.

1¼ cups long-grain brown rice, rinsed and drained

½ medium yellow onion, cut into ¼-inch dice (about 1 cup)

6 medium garlic cloves, minced (about 1 tablespoon)

1 teaspoon dried oregano (preferably Mexican oregano)

2 cups fresh or frozen corn (from about 2 large cobs)

1 medium poblano chile (or green bell pepper), cored, seeded, and cut into ½-inch dice (about 1 cup)

1 medium red bell pepper, cored, seeded, and cut into ½-inch dice (about 1 cup)

1 tablespoon fresh lime juice

2 tablespoons finely chopped fresh cilantro

Sea salt

1. Combine the rice, onion, garlic, and oregano in a large sauté pan over medium-low heat and cook without water for 10 minutes, stirring frequently, to soften the onion and toast the rice. (Do not add any water; there will be enough water from the onion and rinsed rice to prevent burning.)

2. Meanwhile, combine ½ cup of the corn with 1 cup water in a blender and puree.

3. Add the corn cream to the pan with the rice. Add the poblano pepper, the red bell pepper, the remaining corn, and 1 cup water. Bring the liquid to a boil over high heat. Reduce the heat to medium-low, cover, and simmer for 25 to 30 minutes, until the rice is cooked and the water is absorbed. Turn off the heat and let the rice rest, covered, for 10 minutes.

4. Uncover the pan and add the lime juice, cilantro, and salt to taste. Use a fork to fluff the rice and combine the ingredients.

STORAGE: Refrigerate in an airtight container for up to 4 days.

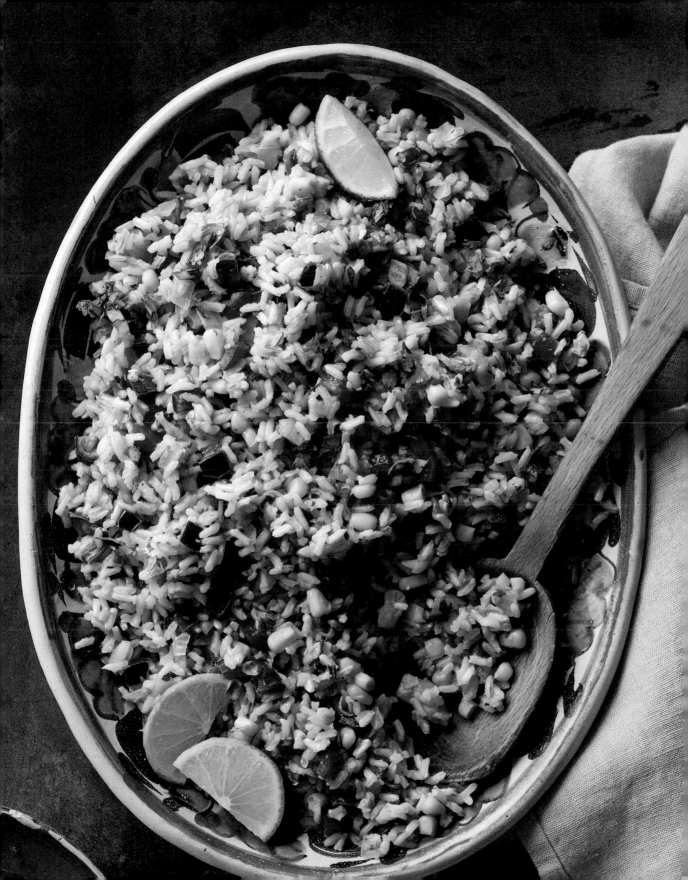

You owe yourself the treat of baking your own bread, at least once in a while. The warm, yeasty scent of baking bread and the experience of breaking into a warm loaf are the epitome of good living.

---

10 | Bread and Crackers

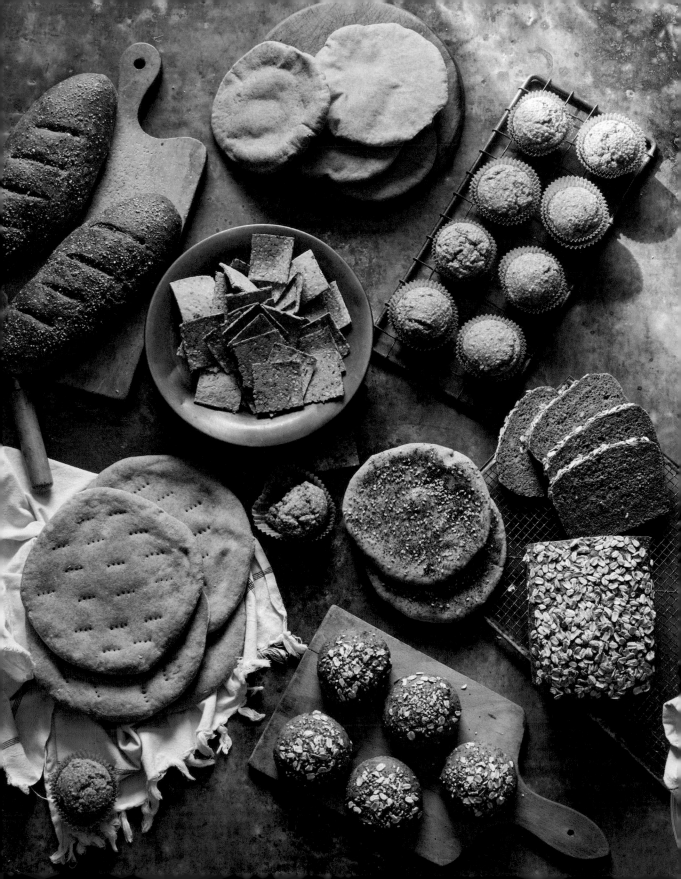

Multigrain Sweet Potato Rolls

These are my version of small, seeded German rolls called *brotchen*. The sweet potato puree keeps the rolls light in texture and adds an earthy, sweet flavor. Multigrain bran is a medley of bran and grits of different grains; you can replace it with rolled oats or cornmeal.

Makes 10 rolls

Ready in 2½ hours

NOTE: You can bake this dough into baguettes or a loaf of sandwich bread. To make baguettes, form the dough into two 9-inch-long logs and place them side by side on a baking sheet. To make a sandwich-size loaf for slicing, put the dough into a 9-by-5-inch silicone or nonstick loaf pan. In either case, the baking temperature and time will be the same as for the rolls.

For the Dough
2 tablespoons pumpkin seeds

2 tablespoons sunflower seeds

¼ cup plus 2 tablespoons hot (but not boiling) water

1 tablespoon Date Paste (page 30; or maple syrup)

1 (¼-ounce) package active dry yeast (approximately 2¼ teaspoons)

1½ cups whole-wheat flour

1½ cups unbleached all-purpose flour (or whole-wheat flour), plus more for dusting

1 (15-ounce) can sweet potato (or pumpkin) puree (about 1⅓ cups)

½ cup multigrain bran

½ teaspoon salt (optional)

For the Topping
½ cup unsweetened, unflavored plant milk

1 tablespoon flaxseed meal (brown or golden)

2 tablespoons rolled oats

1 teaspoon sesame seeds

1 teaspoon poppy seeds

1 teaspoon flaxseeds

1. To make the dough, preheat the oven to 375°F. Line a quarter sheet pan (9 by 13 inches; or a similar-sized baking dish) with parchment paper.

2. Soak the pumpkin and sunflower seeds in ¼ cup of the hot water for 20 minutes.

3. Pour the remaining 2 tablespoons hot water into a food processor fitted with the dough blade or the bowl of a stand mixer fitted with the dough blade. Add the date paste and yeast. Cover and set aside in a warm place for 10 minutes, or until frothy.

4. Drain the seeds and add them to the food processor or mixer bowl. Add the whole-wheat flour, all-purpose flour, sweet potato puree, bran, and salt (if you're using it). If you are using a food processor, run the machine on low speed for 2 minutes

to knead the dough. If you are using a stand mixer, mix with the dough hook on low speed for 2 minutes to knead the dough.

5. If you are using a food processor, dust the bottom of a large bowl with all-purpose flour and transfer the dough to the bowl. Leave the dough in the bowl if you are using a stand mixer. Cover the bowl with a damp cloth and set aside in a warm place for about 1 hour, until the dough has risen to double its size.

6. Dust your work surface and baking sheet lightly with all-purpose flour. Place the dough on the dusted surface and knead it a few times. Divide the dough into 10 equal portions. Roll each portion into a ball and place the balls on the prepared baking sheet, leaving an even amount of space between them. Cover the rolls with the damp cloth and set aside in a warm place for about 30 minutes, until they double in size.

7. Meanwhile, to make the topping, bring the milk to a boil over high heat. Turn off the heat and add the flaxseed meal. Set aside for 10 minutes. Pass the liquid through a strainer, reserving the liquid and discarding the solids to create a "wash."

8. Combine the oats, sesame seeds, poppy seeds, and flaxseeds together in a small bowl.

9. Brush the rolls with the flax wash and sprinkle with the topping mixture.

10. Bake the rolls in the oven for about 40 minutes, until they are crispy and golden brown. Remove from the oven. Serve warm or at room temperature.

STORAGE: Wrap the rolls tightly (or put them in a sealable plastic bag) and store at room temperature for up to 5 days or freeze for up to 1 month.

> "To get the right temperature of warm water, mix half room-temperature and half boiling water. This gives you the right temperature for activating yeast. I figured this out through trial and error, and it has always worked for me."

Za'atar Spiced Pita Bread

Making your own pita bread is much easier than you might think, and even for those of us who live in places where we have access to whole-grain pita bread, there is still a reason to try it. Who doesn't enjoy the smell of the bread baking? It's also fun to watch it puff up in the oven. I give you instructions to make these two ways: as pita breads or, slightly larger, as pizza crusts. The pita are seasoned with za'atar, a popular Middle Eastern spice blend consisting of dried thyme and sumac, sesame seeds, salt, and other spices. I smear tahini on the bread to adhere the spices, but you can use water if you prefer.

Makes 10 pita breads or 6 8-inch pizza crusts

Ready in 2 hours, 40 minutes

1 tablespoon Date Paste (page 30; or maple syrup)

2 teaspoons active dry yeast

2 cups whole-wheat flour

1½ cups unbleached all-purpose flour, plus more for dusting

1 teaspoon sea salt

2 tablespoons tahini (sesame paste; omit if you are making pizza crust)

1 recipe Za'atar Spice (recipe follows)

NOTE: You can use this dough to make pizza crusts. Divide the dough into 6 rounds instead of 10 and roll them out as you do the pita. Poke each round with the tines of a fork and bake them for 6 to 8 minutes. Remove them from the oven, top as desired, and bake for an additional 20 minutes.

1. Preheat the oven to 400°F. Line 2 large baking sheets with parchment paper.

2. Combine the date paste, yeast, and 1½ cups lukewarm water in a food processor fitted with the dough blade or the bowl of a standing mixer fitted with the dough hook. Cover and set aside in a warm place for 10 minutes, or until frothy.

3. Combine the whole-wheat flour, all-purpose flour, and salt in a large mixing bowl. Add the dry ingredients to the food processor or mixer bowl and mix on medium-low speed for 2 to 3 minutes, until the dough begins to pull away from the sides of the bowl. If you used a food processor, transfer the dough to a large mixing bowl. There's no need to transfer the dough if you made it in the bowl of a stand mixer. Cover the bowl with a clean damp cloth. Set aside in a warm place for 45 minutes to 1 hour, until the dough has doubled in size.

4. Lightly dust a large cutting board or another flat work surface with all-purpose flour. Scrape the dough out of the bowl onto the dusted surface and knead for about 1 minute. Return it to the bowl, cover with the cloth, and set it in a warm place again to rise for another 30 minutes.

5. Meanwhile, make the za'atar spice according to the recipe below.

6. Divide the dough into 10 equal portions. Dust your hands and the dough with flour and roll each portion into a ball. Dust a flat work surface and rolling pin with flour. Roll each ball of dough into a 6-inch round. Transfer the dough rounds to the prepared baking sheets, placing an equal number of rounds on each.

7. Loosely cover the dough with clean damp towels and set near the stove to rise for 10 minutes.

8. Place the pita in the oven and bake for 4 to 6 minutes, until the undersides are golden. Remove from the oven and use a spatula to turn each of them around.

9. Use the back of a spoon to spread a thin layer of tahini on each pita and sprinkle with the za'atar spice, dividing it evenly. Return to the oven and bake for 4 to 6 minutes, until the dough puffs up.

10. Remove from the oven and set aside until cool enough to handle. Serve warm or at room temperature.

STORAGE: Place a sheet of wax paper between each piece of bread to prevent them from sticking together. Wrap the pita tightly in plastic (or put them into a sealable plastic bag) and store at room temperature for up to 5 days or freeze for up to 1 month.

Za'atar Spice

Makes about ½ cup	3 tablespoons sesame seeds	1 tablespoon dried thyme	Sea salt to taste
Ready in 5 minutes	2 tablespoons dried sumac	1 tablespoon garlic powder	Freshly ground black pepper to taste

Combine all the ingredients in a small bowl and whisk well to blend. Store in an airtight container at room temperature indefinitely.

Double Corn Muffins

These corn muffins contain mashed corn kernels along with cornmeal, so they are very moist and flavorful. Serve them as a snack, smeared with date paste or tahini, or alongside soup, such as Louisiana Vegetable Gumbo (page 199) or Caldo Verde: Portuguese Potato and Kale Soup (page 206). When I make these, I make a double batch. I keep a few fresh to eat right away, and I freeze the rest to warm up when I want them.

Makes 12 muffins

Ready in 1 hour, 10 minutes

2 cups fresh or frozen corn kernels (from about 2 large cobs)

1 cup unsweetened, unflavored plant milk

¼ cup plus 2 tablespoons pure maple syrup

1 tablespoon flaxseed meal (brown or golden)

1¼ cups whole-wheat flour

1 cup coarse cornmeal (or polenta)

½ cup almond flour

2 teaspoons baking powder

½ teaspoon sea salt

NOTE: You will need a standard-size muffin pan to make this.

1. Preheat the oven to 350°F. Line a muffin pan with liners.

2. Combine the corn, milk, maple syrup, and flaxseed meal in a food processor and blend until the corn kernels are coarsely chopped. Add the whole-wheat flour, cornmeal, almond flour, baking powder, and salt and process until the wet and dry ingredients are combined.

3. Spoon the batter into the muffin cups, dividing it evenly. Bake the muffins in the oven for 35 to 40 minutes, until a toothpick inserted in the middle of a muffin comes out clean. Remove the muffin pan from the oven and place it on a rack to cool for 5 to 10 minutes. Remove the muffins from the pan and place them on the rack to cool completely.

STORAGE: Wrap the muffins tightly in plastic (or put them in a sealable plastic bag) and store at room temperature for up to 5 days or freeze for up to 1 month.

Dessert is the very embodiment of indulgence. It is a pleasure to be savored and enjoyed in small quantities. Take it as a metaphor for life: slow down and appreciate every bite.

---

11 | Desserts

Mini Parisian Fruit Tarts

Makes 24
bite-size tarts

Ready in 1 hour

I love the pretty fruit tarts you see in French bakeries and the way in which the fruit is arranged so nicely on them. I make the creamy filling for these two-bite tarts from pureed winter squash. The crust, made from sorghum flour and ground walnuts, is gluten-free. The tarts make a satisfying afternoon sweet and an easy-to-eat dessert for entertaining. You'll have more filling than you need for the tarts; I use it as I would apple butter, spread on toast or spooned over pancakes, waffles, or French toast. To make this recipe even easier than it already is, start with peeled, cut-up squash.

NOTE: You will need a silicone or nonstick mini cupcake pan to make these.

For the Filling
1 medium acorn squash, peeled and cut into 1-inch dice (about 5 cups)

1 tablespoon pure maple syrup

1 teaspoon orange zest

Pinch of saffron (optional)

For the Crust
1¼ cups old-fashioned rolled oats

¾ cup walnuts

¾ cup sorghum flour (or whole-wheat flour), plus more as needed

Pinch of sea salt

½ cup pure maple syrup

2 teaspoons pure vanilla extract

For the Topping
2 cups berries or diced or sliced fruit

1. To make the filling, place a steamer basket in a medium saucepan and add 1 to 2 inches of water to the pan. Bring the water to a simmer over medium-high heat. Place the acorn squash in the steamer, cover, and steam until tender when pierced with a fork, 15 to 20 minutes. Turn off the heat, uncover the saucepan, and set aside to cool to room temperature.

2. Transfer the squash to a blender. Add the maple syrup, orange zest, and saffron (if you're using it) and blend until smooth. Refrigerate, covered, until you are ready to assemble the tarts or for up to 2 days.

3. To make the crust, preheat the oven to 350°F.

4. Combine the oats, walnuts, flour, and salt in a food processor fitted with a metal

blade and grind to a fine meal. Add the maple syrup and vanilla extract and pulse until the mixture starts to bind. The mixture should be crumbly, but it should bind when pinched between your fingers.

5. Drop 1 tablespoon of the crust mixture into each cupcake cup and press to line the bottom and sides of the cup evenly. (If the mixture is too sticky to handle, dip your fingers in water or flour and continue.)

6. Bake the crusts in the oven until they are light brown and crisp, 20 to 30 minutes. Remove from the oven and set aside to cool to room temperature.

7. Spoon 1 heaping teaspoon of the filling into each tart and use the top of the spoon to smooth it out. Arrange the fruit on top of the tarts and put the tarts on a platter or baking sheet. Serve immediately, or cover with plastic wrap and refrigerate until you are ready to serve.

STORAGE: Cover and refrigerate for up to 3 days.

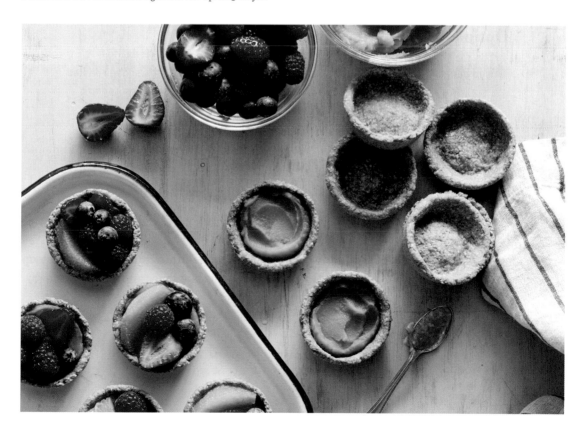

"Cooking yams with the skin prevents them from getting too watery."

1. To make the crust, preheat the oven to 350°F. Line the bottom of a springform pan with parchment paper.

2. Combine the flour, walnuts, sugar, flaxseed meal, baking powder, cinnamon, and salt in a food processor and blend to grind the nuts and combine the ingredients. Add 2 tablespoons water and pulse to incorporate. The mixture will be crumbly, but it should bind when pinched between your fingers. If it doesn't, add another tablespoon of water and pulse to combine.

3. Spoon the crust mixture into the prepared cake pan. Use the bottom of a bowl or a ladle to press it in evenly, forming an even crust. Bake the crust in the oven for 20 minutes. Remove the crust from the oven and place it on a cooling rack to cool to room temperature.

4. Meanwhile, to make the filling, place a steamer basket in a medium saucepan and add 1 to 2 inches of water to the pan. Bring the water to a simmer over medium-high heat. Place the yams in the steamer, cover, and steam until tender when pierced with a fork, about 30 minutes. Uncover and place the yams under running water to cool. Slip off and discard the peels. Transfer the yams to a bowl and mash them lightly.

5. Transfer the mashed yams to a food processor. Add the milk, sugar, lime juice, and lime zest and process until smooth.

6. Spoon the filling into the prepared crust and use a spatula to spread it out evenly. Place the pie in the refrigerator to chill for at least 1 hour.

7. To make the sauce, combine the blueberries, sugar, and 3 tablespoons water in a small saucepan and bring to a boil over high heat. Reduce the heat to low and simmer for about 3 minutes, until the blueberries begin to break down and the liquid is syrupy. Turn off the heat and stir in the lime zest.

8. To serve, remove the sides of the springform pan from the pie. Slice and drizzle the sauce on top.

STORAGE: Cover and refrigerate for up to 5 days.

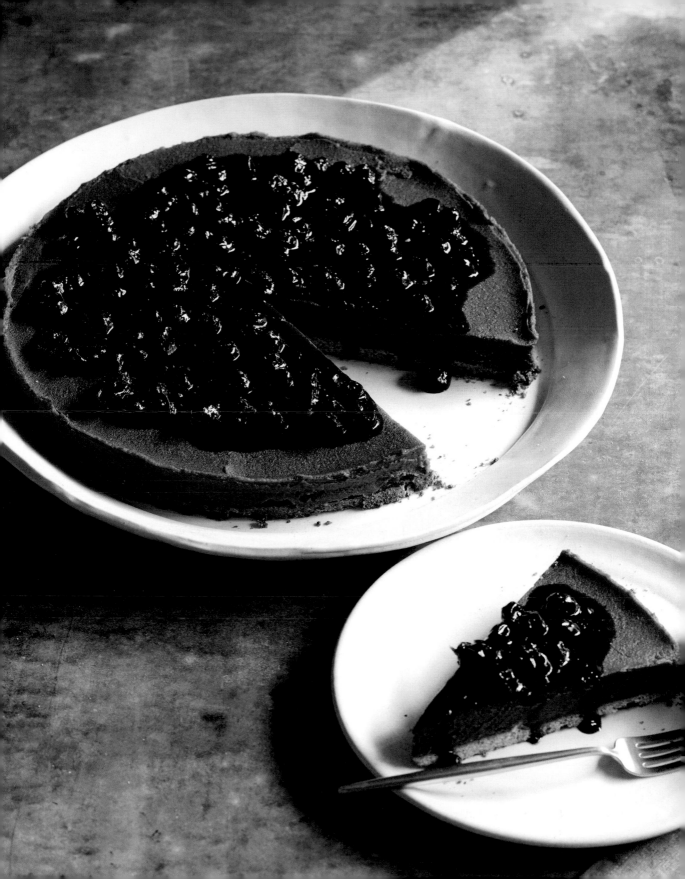

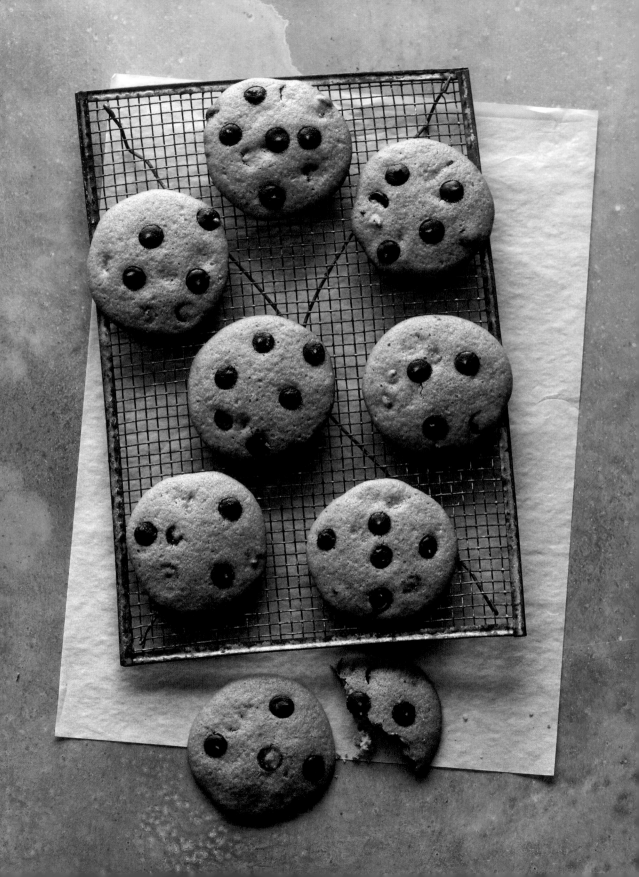

Gerry's Chocolate Chip Cookies

Brian's father, Gerry, loves chocolate chip cookies, and he is very specific about how he wants them: crispy all over and with lots of chocolate chips. I made these especially for him, and now our family bond is stronger than ever. Made with oat flour, the cookies are gluten-free.

Makes 16 to 18 cookies

Ready in 1 hour

NOTE: I use whole cane sugar in this recipe, which enables the cookies to get crisp. If you substitute maple syrup or date sugar for the cane sugar, the cookies will still be delicious, but they won't have the same appealing crunch.

1½ cups oat flour	⅔ cup whole cane sugar	3 tablespoons almond butter (or tahini)
1 tablespoon arrowroot powder	⅓ cup unsweetened, unflavored plant milk	1 teaspoon pure vanilla extract
2 teaspoons baking powder	¼ cup unsweetened applesauce	¾ cup grain-sweetened vegan chocolate chips
½ teaspoon sea salt		

1. Preheat the oven to 325°F. Line 2 large baking sheets with parchment paper.

2. Stir the flour, arrowroot, baking powder, and salt in a large mixing bowl to thoroughly combine. In another large mixing bowl, combine the sugar, milk, applesauce, almond butter, and vanilla and whisk to combine.

3. Add the dry mixture to the bowl with the plant milk and sugar mixture and stir until no flour is visible. Stir in the chocolate chips.

4. Drop the cookie dough onto the prepared baking sheets in 2 tablespoon–size balls, leaving at least 1½ inches between them.

5. Bake the cookies in the oven for 40 minutes, or until they are lightly browned but still soft to the touch; they will crisp up once removed from the oven. (For extra-crunchy cookies, bake for another 10 minutes.)

6. Remove the cookies from the oven and let them cool for 5 minutes. Transfer the cookies to a cooling rack to cool completely.

STORAGE: Store in an airtight container or sealable plastic bag at room temperature for up to 10 days or freeze for up to 1 month.

4. Lightly dust your work surface or cutting board with all-purpose flour. Transfer the dough to the floured surface and knead for a few minutes until the dough is smooth. Divide the dough into 8 equal portions and roll each portion into a ball with your hands.

5. To assemble the hand pies, prepare an assembly line including a rolling pin, a pastry brush, and a bowl containing all-purpose flour for dusting. Clear a clean, flat work surface or cutting board for rolling out the dough.

6. Dust a rolling pin with flour and roll one ball of dough into an 8-inch disk, dusting the work surface and dough with flour as needed. With a knife or bench scraper, trim off the edges to cut the disk to form a square. Reserve the scraps to reroll.

7. Divide the square of dough into four imaginary quadrants. Mound 2 tablespoons of the filling in each of the two lower quadrants. Fold the top edge of the dough to meet the bottom edge, covering the filling and forming a rectangle with the long edge facing you. Using a bench scraper or knife, cut the rectangle in half down the middle to form two hand pies. Press on the edges of the dough with the tines of a fork or your fingertips to seal the edges, dusting your fingers or the fork with flour if the dough is too sticky to crimp. Transfer the finished hand pies to one of the prepared baking sheets.

8. Repeat, rolling out the remaining dough and filling, cutting and crimping them as you did the first batch, placing them on the second prepared baking sheet as they are completed. Reroll the reserved scraps to form additional hand pies.

9. Place both baking sheets in the oven and bake the hand pies for 25 minutes.

10. Meanwhile, combine the flaxseed meal in a small bowl with ½ cup hot water and let stand for 10 minutes. Strain, reserving the liquid, and discard the contents of the strainer.

11. Remove the hand pies from the oven and increase the oven temperature to 400°F.

12. Brush each hand pie with the flaxseed gel and sprinkle liberally with sugar. Return the hand pies to the oven, rotating them from front to back and top to bottom rack and bake for about 5 minutes, until they are golden brown.

13. Remove the hand pies from the oven. Allow them to cool for at least 5 minutes before serving. Serve warm or at room temperature.

STORAGE: Place in a covered container or sealable plastic bag and refrigerate for up to 4 days or freeze for up to 1 month.

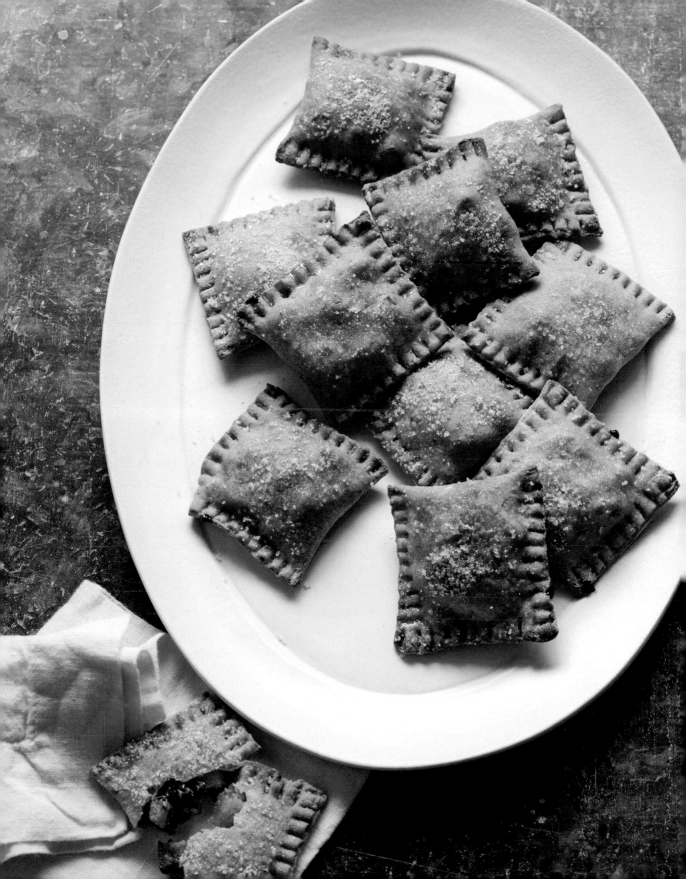

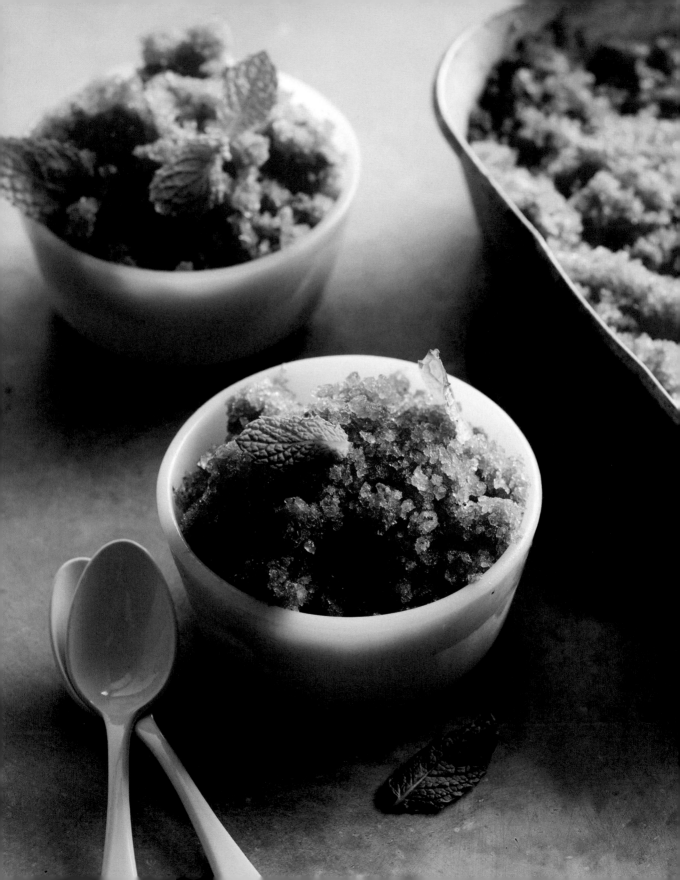

Lemon-Watermelon Granita

Granita, Italian shaved ice, is the ultimate summertime dessert. This one is made with the refreshing combination of watermelon, lemon, and mint.

Makes about
4 cups

Ready in 1 hour, 10 minutes (or about 4 hours if you are not using an ice cream machine)

1 cup plus 2 tablespoons apple juice

¼ cup pure maple syrup

2 tablespoons arrowroot powder

6 cups chopped, seeded watermelon (about 1¾ pounds)

⅓ cup fresh mint leaves, plus more for garnish

2 tablespoons fresh lemon juice

1. Combine 1 cup of the apple juice and the maple syrup in a small saucepan and bring to a boil over high heat. Reduce the heat to medium and simmer for about 10 minutes, until the liquid has reduced to about 1 cup. (I do this by sight, but if you want to be especially careful, you can pour it into a measuring cup.)

2. Meanwhile, in a small bowl, use a fork to mix the arrowroot with the remaining 2 tablespoons apple juice until no lumps remain. (This mixture is called a slurry.) Add the slurry to the saucepan with the juice. Reduce the heat to medium and cook until the mixture is thick and gummy, about 1 minute. Turn off the heat and let the mixture cool to room temperature.

3. Combine the watermelon, mint leaves, lemon juice, and thickened juice mixture in a blender and puree until smooth.

4. To make the granita in an ice cream maker, pour the liquid into an ice cream maker and churn for 20 to 30 minutes, until the mix forms a creamy sorbetlike texture. Serve immediately or transfer to a covered container and freeze until ready to serve. To make the granita without an ice cream maker, pour the watermelon mixture into a 9-by-12-inch baking dish and place in the freezer until it is solid, 4 to 5 hours. Remove the dish from the freezer and let it sit at room temperature for about 5 minutes to soften. To serve, scrape the granita with a fork to form crystals, and scoop the crystals into serving glasses or into a storage container.

5. Garnish each serving with fresh mint leaves.

STORAGE: Freeze in a covered container for up to 2 weeks.

5. To assemble the baklava, warm the syrup over low heat if necessary. Create an assembly line of the tortilla disks, filling, syrup, and individual serving bowls. Drop the disks into the syrup and let them sit for 1 to 2 minutes to absorb the syrup. Spoon 1 tablespoon of the syrup and place one disk in the bottom of each serving bowl. Spoon 1 tablespoon of the nut filling onto each disk. Place another tortilla in each bowl and repeat with the filling until you have 4 disks in each bowl. Top each serving with a sprinkling of the filling on the top and a drizzle of the warm syrup. Serve right away.

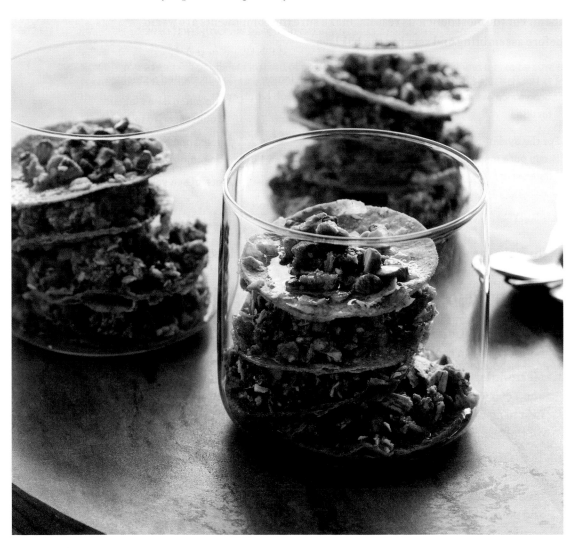

Kesar-Pista Kulfi: Saffron Pistachio "Ice Cream"

One of my best childhood memories is of going for evening walks in the summertime with my family in the local park in Mumbai, where I grew up. My parents would treat my siblings and me to kulfi, India's dense, creamy version of ice cream, on which this recipe is based. "Kesar-pista" or saffron-pistachio is one of the most popular flavors of kulfi. This recipe gets its creaminess from white yams. A little bit of fresh spinach gives the ice cream a bright pistachio color.

NOTE: You will need a 9-by-5-inch silicone or nonstick loaf pan to make this.

Makes about
3 cups

Ready in 4½ hours

12 ounces white yams, peeled and cut into 1-inch pieces (about 3 cups)

½ cup roasted, shelled pistachios

¾ cup unsweetened, unflavored plant milk

¾ cup fresh spinach (about 1 ounce)

⅓ cup pure maple syrup

½ teaspoon ground cardamom

Pinch of saffron

1. If you are using a nonstick loaf pan rather than a silicone loaf pan, line the bottom with plastic wrap.

2. Place a steamer basket in a medium saucepan and add 1 to 2 inches of water to the pan. Bring the water to a simmer over medium-high heat. Place the yams in the steamer, cover, and steam until tender when pierced with a fork, 20 minutes. Remove the lid and set aside to cool to room temperature.

3. Place the pistachios on a dish towel, close the towel, and rub to remove as much of the skins as possible. Discard the skins and put the pistachios into a food processor. Pulse to chop coarsely. Set aside 2 tablespoons of the pistachios and leave the rest in the food processor. Add the yams, milk, spinach, maple syrup, cardamom, and saffron and blend until smooth and creamy.

4. Sprinkle the reserved pistachios to cover the bottom of the loaf pan. Spoon the kulfi mixture over the pistachios. Cover the pan with plastic wrap and chill the kulfi in the freezer for at least 4 hours.

5. When you're ready to serve the kulfi, invert the pan to transfer it to a platter. Dip a sharp knife into hot water and slice the kulfi to the thickness you desire.

STORAGE: Cover and freeze for up to 2 weeks.

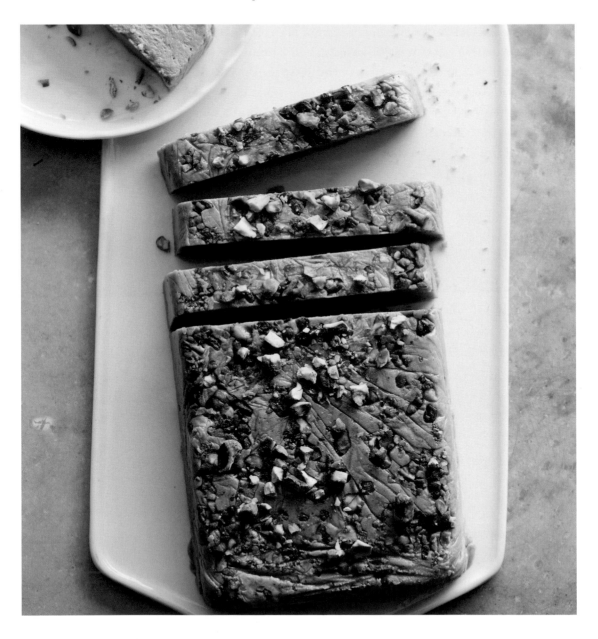

German Marble Cake
with Raspberries

This recipe is inspired by a traditional German cake referred to as "Oma's [Grandma's] marble cake." It is composed of half orange-chocolate cake and half vanilla cake, with raspberries strewn throughout. It took me a long time and a lot of experimenting to create two cakes that had the same texture and required the same baking time, but the results are as pretty as they are delicious. I make this cake with a combination of sorghum and oat flours, which makes it gluten-free. If gluten isn't an issue for you, you can use whole-wheat flour in place of either or both of them.

Makes 1 9-by-5-inch loaf cake

Ready in 1 hour, 10 minutes

NOTE: You will need a 9-by-5-inch silicone or nonstick loaf pan to make this.

1 (12-ounce) package soft silken tofu, drained

¾ cup whole cane sugar

¾ cup sorghum flour (or whole-wheat flour)

¾ cup oat flour (or whole-wheat flour)

2 tablespoons pure vanilla extract

½ tablespoon apple cider vinegar

½ teaspoon baking powder

½ teaspoon baking soda

¼ teaspoon sea salt

¼ cup cocoa powder

2 teaspoons orange extract

½ cup raspberries

1. Preheat the oven to 325°F. Line the bottom and sides of a 9-by-5-inch loaf pan with a piece of parchment paper.

2. Combine the tofu, sugar, sorghum flour, oat flour, vanilla, vinegar, baking powder, baking soda, and salt in a food processor fitted with a metal blade and pulse to form a smooth batter. Transfer 1½ cups of the batter to a large bowl.

3. Add the cocoa powder and orange extract to the batter remaining in the food processor and blend to combine.

4. Pour the chocolate batter into the loaf pan. Pour the reserved vanilla batter over the chocolate batter to cover it completely. Scatter the raspberries on top of the batter and press to submerge them completely. Insert a fork or table knife into the

From baked entrees to simply prepared seasonal vegetables, it's the flavor, texture, and temperature of the right sauce that takes the dish to another level. If you have sauce, you are halfway to a delicious dinner.

12 | Dips and Sauces

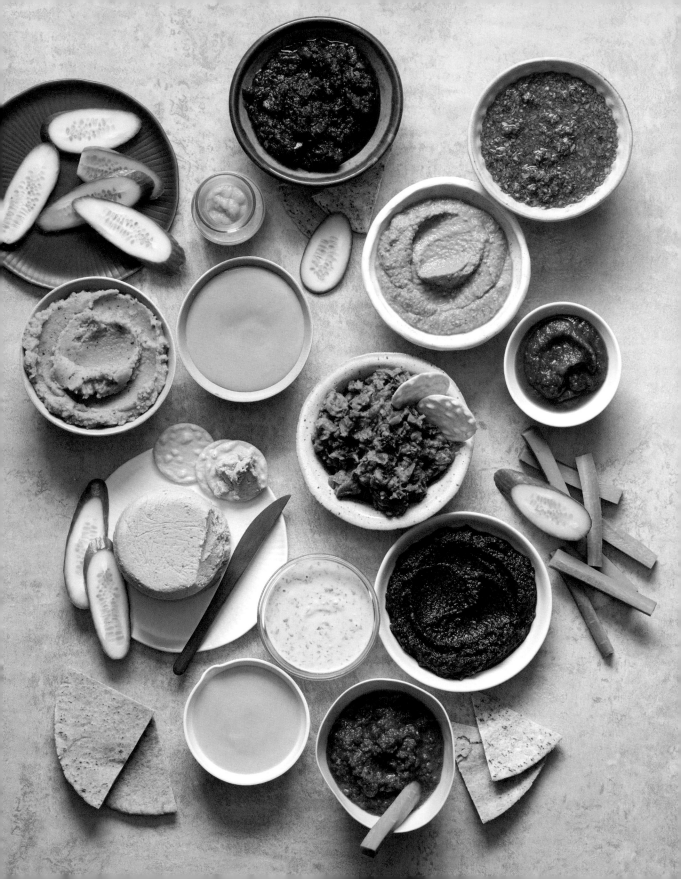

Chipotle Barbecue Sauce

As much as I love all-American tomato-based barbecue sauce, the commercial varieties are too high in added sugar and salt for a whole-food, plant-based diet, so I like to make my own. I use this as a sauce for Texas Toast with Chipotle Barbecue Beans (page 51) and also to toss with Buffalo Cauliflower Bites (page 79).

Makes about
2 cups

Ready in
15 minutes

½ cup grape or apple juice

½ cup tomato paste

¼ cup white wine vinegar

¼ cup whole cane sugar (or Date Paste, page 30)

2 tablespoons garlic powder

2 tablespoons onion powder

1 tablespoon arrowroot powder

½ tablespoon smoked sweet paprika

½ teaspoon dried celery stalk (optional; available in the spice section of specialty food stores)

½ chipotle chile in adobo sauce, finely chopped

Pinch of mustard powder

Combine all the ingredients in a medium saucepan. Add 1½ cups water and bring to a boil over high heat. Reduce the heat to medium-low and simmer the sauce for 10 minutes to meld the flavors. Use as is, or strain if you prefer a smoother sauce.

STORAGE: Cool the sauce to room temperature. Transfer to a container with a tight-fitting lid and refrigerate for up to 1 week.

Tofu "Sour Cream"

Makes about
1½ cups

Ready in 5 minutes

This condiment is simple to make, and it's delicious spooned on soup, potato pancakes, baked potatoes, and, of course, any Mexican dish such as tacos or tostadas. I call for it in the following recipes: Crunchy Hash Brown Waffles with Applesauce (page 52), Black Bean Chilaquiles with Fire-Roasted Tomatillo Salsa (page 63), and Dutch Potato and Apple Salad (page 123), as well as on Huaraches: Mexican Masa "Flatbreads" with Beans and Lime-Spiked Salad (page 134).

1 (12-ounce) package extra-firm tofu, drained

3 tablespoons fresh lemon juice

1 tablespoon white wine vinegar

½ teaspoon sea salt

¼ teaspoon yellow mustard

Blend all the ingredients in a blender until pureed.

STORAGE: Refrigerate in a container with a tight-fitting lid for up to 1 week.

Chipotle "Sour Cream"

Chipotle chiles in adobo sauce come in a small can and can be found in the Hispanic section of supermarkets. The adobo sauce they are packed in has so much flavor, I use it to give a sweet smoky flavor (and heat) to this "sour cream." I like to spoon it on soups, tacos, tostadas, or anything else with a Mexican touch. It is an integral component of the Lentil Tacos with Chipotle "Sour Cream" (page 144) and Salvadoran Breakfast Tortillas with Chipotle "Sour Cream" (page 41).

Makes about
1½ cups

Ready in 5 minutes

1 (12-ounce) package extra-firm tofu, drained

¼ cup fresh lime juice

¼ cup chipotle juice (from a can of chipotles in adobo sauce)

1 medium garlic clove, minced (about ¼ teaspoon)

Pinch of sea salt

Blend all the ingredients in a blender until pureed.

STORAGE: Refrigerate in a container with a tight-fitting lid for up to 1 week.

Fire-Roasted Tomatillo Salsa

Makes about
2 cups

Ready in
35 minutes

The ingredients of this salsa are roasted over high heat, so they get a nice smoky flavor that you really taste. I call for you to do this under the broiler, but you could also cook them on an outdoor grill. I use it to make the Black Bean Chilaquiles with Fire-Roasted Tomatillo Salsa (page 63) and to dress Huaraches: Mexican Masa "Flatbreads" with Beans and Lime-Spiked Salad (page 134).

1 pound tomatillos, husks removed

½ (15-ounce) can sodium-free or low-sodium diced tomatoes (about 1½ cups; preferably fire-roasted)

1 poblano pepper, stem removed (about 2½ ounces)

½ small yellow onion, cut into large pieces (about ½ cup)

2 medium garlic cloves, minced (about 1 teaspoon)

4 or 5 fresh cilantro sprigs

½ teaspoon dried oregano (preferably Mexican oregano)

½ teaspoon ground cumin

Sea salt

Freshly ground black pepper

1. Preheat the broiler. Put the tomatillos, tomatoes, poblano pepper, onion, and garlic onto a baking sheet and place them under the broiler for 30 minutes, or until they are charred slightly. Set aside to cool slightly.

2. Transfer the contents of the baking sheet to a blender, add the cilantro, oregano, and cumin, and puree. Season with salt and pepper to taste.

STORAGE: Refrigerate in an airtight container for up to 1 week.

Peanut Sauce

This sauce is my quick, easy, low-fat version of traditional Thai peanut sauce. It calls for no hard-to-find ingredients, and it comes together in minutes. I drizzle it on Thai Quinoa Salad with Peanut Sauce (page 277), and I serve it as a dip with Vietnamese Summer Rolls (page 153).

Makes about 1 cup

Ready in 5 minutes

⅓ cup peanut butter

2 tablespoons fresh lemon juice

1 tablespoon sriracha

1 tablespoon pure maple syrup

1 garlic clove, minced (about ½ teaspoon)

Sea salt

Combine the peanut butter, lemon juice, sriracha, maple syrup, and garlic in a blender. Add ½ cup water and blend to a smooth consistency. Add salt to taste and pulse to distribute it.

STORAGE: Refrigerate in an airtight container for up to 1 week.

Fresh Cilantro Chutney

Makes about 1 cup

Ready in
10 minutes

This chutney uses a lot of cilantro, as well as a lot of other vegetables. If you want to make it as spicy as traditional Indian chutney, use twice as much jalapeño. You can replace the mango with another tropical fruit, such as pineapple, guava, or passion fruit. Serve it as a dipping sauce with Sweet Potato Tikkis with Fresh Cilantro Chutney (page 75) and Punjabi Samosas (page 93), and on Brian's Indian Burritos with Fresh Cilantro Chutney (page 145).

2 packed cups fresh cilantro leaves and stems

½ medium tomato, roughly chopped (about ½ cup)

1 celery stalk, roughly chopped (about ⅓ cup)

1 medium shallot (about 2 ounces), roughly chopped

¼ cup fresh or frozen mango (about 1½ ounces)

1 jalapeño pepper, seeded

1 tablespoon fresh lemon juice

1 (½-inch) piece peeled fresh ginger

1 small garlic clove

Combine the ingredients in a blender and blend to a smooth consistency.

STORAGE: Refrigerate in an airtight container for up to 1 week.

Nepalese Tomato Chutney

I was given this recipe by the same Nepali friend, Reena, who taught me how to make Nepali momos. It is a little different from any chutney I've had in India; it's so simple, with so few ingredients—yet the flavor is so vibrant. Serve it with Reena's Momos with Nepalese Tomato Chutney (page 103) and any other Indian-inspired dishes.

Makes about 1 cup

Ready in
10 minutes

2 medium tomatoes, cut into ¾-inch dice (about 2 cups)	1 tablespoon fresh lemon juice	Sea salt
4 medium garlic cloves, minced (about 2 teaspoons)	2 sprigs fresh cilantro	Freshly ground black pepper

1. Cook the tomato and garlic in a medium sauté pan over medium heat for about 5 minutes, until the tomatoes have broken down and released their juice. Remove from the heat and set aside to cool slightly.

2. Transfer the contents of the pan to a blender. Add the lemon juice, cilantro, and salt and pepper to taste and blend until smooth, adding water 1 to 2 tablespoons at a time to reach a smooth consistency.

STORAGE: Refrigerate in an airtight container for up to 1 week.

Chimichurri

Chimichurri is an Argentinian condiment made by blending fresh herbs and other seasonings—no cooking involved. It's traditionally served as a dipping sauce for empanadas. I sometimes add kale to this recipe, which adds another nice layer of flavor in addition to bulking it up with green vegetables. If you want to try it that way, add 2 leaves of kale, stems removed and discarded, to this recipe. In addition to being a key dipping sauce with Corn and Mushroom Empanadas with Chimichurri (page 69), I brush it on Summer Vegetable Skewers with Chimichurri (page 171). It is also delicious spooned into grain bowls, soups, and salads or as a dipping sauce with tortilla chips or bread.

2½ packed cups fresh curly or flat-leaf parsley leaves and stems

1½ packed cups fresh cilantro leaves and stems

2 tablespoons white wine vinegar

½ tablespoon fresh lemon juice

4 medium garlic cloves

1 jalapeño pepper (if you're using it), seeded

1 teaspoon dried oregano

¼ teaspoon red pepper flakes (optional)

Sea salt to taste

Combine all the ingredients in a food processor. Add ½ cup water and pulse until the herbs are finely chopped, adding more water as necessary to make a loose, spoonable sauce.

STORAGE: Refrigerate in an airtight container for up to 1 week.

Parsley Tahini Sauce

Tahini sauce is easy to make and so flavorful that I always have it in my refrigerator to use as a salad dressing, to spread on toast, or to add a burst of flavor to grain bowls. I add parsley to the classic sauce, which gives it a fresh flavor and pretty color. In place of the parsley in this recipe, you could use fresh cilantro, tarragon, mint, or a combination of these herbs. The sauce is an integral component of the Middle Eastern Pita Pocket Sandwiches (page 159), Zucchini Rollatini Stuffed with Quinoa and Chickpeas (page 232), and Mujadara Bowls with Parsley Tahini Sauce (page 287).

Makes about ½ cup

Ready in
10 minutes

¼ cup tahini (sesame paste)

2 tablespoons fresh lemon juice

2 tablespoons finely chopped fresh parsley

3 medium garlic cloves, minced (about 1½ teaspoons)

Sea salt

Combine the tahini, lemon juice, parsley, and garlic in a medium bowl. Add ¼ cup water and stir until the sauce is creamy and no lumps of tahini remain, adding more water if needed to achieve a drizzling consistency. Add salt to taste.

STORAGE: Refrigerate in a covered container for up to 1 week. The sauce will thicken as it sits, so you may need to stir in a tablespoon or more water before serving.

Four-Chile Salsa

Makes about
2 cups

Ready in
20 minutes

I use a variety of ground chiles in this salsa; each contributes a unique flavor. You could simplify the recipe by using fewer varieties or even just one. It is such a versatile salsa to use as a condiment for anything Mexican, such as Huaraches: Mexican Masa "Flatbreads" with Beans and Lime-Spiked Salad (page 134), Lentil Tacos with Chipotle "Sour Cream" (page 144), Mexican Chopped Salad (page 124), Spinach and "Cheese" Pupusas with Red Cabbage Slaw (page 141), and Smoky Black Bean Nachos (page 87).

1 pound Roma tomatoes, seeded and cut into ¼-inch dice (about 3 cups)

1 serrano chile, seeded (for a very spicy salsa, do not remove the seeds)

4 medium garlic cloves, minced (about 2 teaspoons)

2 teaspoons ancho chile powder

2 teaspoons California chile powder (or New Mexico chile powder)

1 teaspoon guajillo chile powder

¼ small yellow onion, cut into ¼-inch dice (about ¼ cup)

2 tablespoons finely chopped fresh cilantro

2 tablespoons fresh lime juice

Sea salt

1. Put 2 cups of the chopped tomatoes into a medium saucepan. Add the serrano chile, garlic, ancho chile powder, California chile powder, and guajillo chile powder. Cook over high heat until the tomatoes begin to bubble. Reduce the heat to low and simmer for 10 minutes to meld the flavors. Turn off the heat and set the salsa aside to cool slightly.

2. Transfer the contents of the saucepan to a blender or food processor and blend until smooth. Transfer the salsa to a medium bowl. Add the onion, cilantro, lime juice, and the remaining tomatoes and stir to combine. Add salt to taste.

STORAGE: Refrigerate in an airtight container for up to 1 week.

Gochujang

Gochujang is a red pepper paste traditionally used in Korean cuisine. Commercial versions are too high in added sugar and salt for my taste and also often too spicy. I make my own so I can control these three elements. I use gochujang as a dressing for the Crunchy Vegetable Salad with Korean Hot Sauce (page 117) and as a condiment for the Bibimbap: Korean Rice Bowl (page 272).

Makes about ½ cup

Ready in 5 minutes

½ cup applesauce

1 tablespoon tomato paste

1 teaspoon sriracha

½ medium garlic clove, minced (about ¼ teaspoon)

Stir the ingredients together to combine.

STORAGE: Refrigerate in an airtight container for up to 1 week.

Harissa

Makes about 1 cup

Ready in
10 minutes

I love the intense flavors of harissa, a spicy paste made with fresh chiles, bell peppers, garlic, and dry spices such as cumin, coriander, and chile powder, that is common in many different North African cuisines. (Harissa is also sold as a blend of dry spices.) My recipe differs from those you find in stores in that it is oil-free and low in sodium. I use it in the Tunisian Couscous and Carrot Salad (page 128) and the Harissa Hummus (page 72), and it is an optional condiment to serve with the Mujadara Bowls with Parsley Tahini Sauce (page 287). I also spoon it into soups, stews, and pasta dishes.

½ cup jarred roasted red bell pepper

2 tablespoons tomato paste

2 tablespoons finely chopped fresh mint (or 1 tablespoon dried)

2 tablespoons California chile powder (or smoked paprika)

9 medium garlic cloves, minced (about 1½ tablespoons)

1 tablespoon fresh lemon juice

1 teaspoon ground caraway

½ teaspoon ground coriander

½ teaspoon ground cumin

¼ teaspoon árbol chile powder (or cayenne), plus more to taste

1 teaspoon fresh lemon juice

Sea salt

1. Combine all the ingredients except the lemon juice and salt in a small sauté pan. Add ½ cup water and stir to break up the tomato paste. Cook over medium heat for about 5 minutes, until the sauce thickens.

2. Transfer the sauce to a mini food processor or blender, add the lemon juice, and blend into a smooth paste. Add salt to taste and set aside to cool to room temperature.

STORAGE: Store in a jar with a tight-fitting lid for up to 1 week.

Acknowledgments

First of all, I would like to thank my beloved, Brian Wendel, for loving me, for being the biggest fan of my food, for having introduced me to the whole-food, plant-based lifestyle, and for including me in his life's mission of spreading the message of food being the source for healing and good health.

I would also like to thank my mother, Jaywanti Thacker, for teaching me the secrets of Indian cuisine, for inspiring me through her adventurous and passionate cooking, and for taking so much joy in preparing meals for the family.

Thank you, Carolynn Carreño, for putting my stories and ideas into words, for sharing your valuable knowledge of food, and for being so helpful with your constructive feedback.

Thank you, Josie Bonilla, for being the best support one can ask for in a kitchen, for keeping me on track with deadlines, taking meticulous notes, and making the recipe testing go smoothly by always being prepared.

Thank you, Janis Donnaud, for guiding and championing this cookbook from inception, and for your advice through every step of the production.

Thank you, Karen Rinaldi and the Harper Wave team, for the opportunity to share my recipes with readers, and for your hard work in designing, editing, and distributing this book.

Thank you, Matt Armendariz, Adam Pierson, and Byron Gamarro for the beautiful photography and for being so much fun to work with.

And last but not the least, I thank my family, friends, and the Forks Over Knives team, who have supported me every step of the way, and helped me fine-tune my recipes with their willingness to taste dishes (again and again) and provide valuable insights.

Index

Page numbers of photographs appear in italics.

About the Author

DARSHANA THACKER is chef and culinary project manager for Forks Over Knives and a graduate of the Natural Gourmet Institute in New York City. Darshana grew up cooking alongside her mother and aunts in her native India, and today draws inspiration from cuisines around the world. She's known for her hearty and distinctly flavorful creations, which come from a wide range of ethnic traditions. Chef Darshana was the recipe author of *Forks Over Knives Family* and a lead recipe contributor for the *New York Times* bestseller *The Forks Over Knives Plan*. Her recipes have been published in *The Prevent and Reverse Heart Disease Cookbook*; *Forks Over Knives—The Cookbook*; *Forks Over Knives: The Plant-Based Way to Health*; and *LA Yoga* magazine online. Chef Darshana has catered numerous events, served as a private chef, and regularly holds individual and group cooking classes.